# Natural
# Solutions
## *for*
# Pain-Free
# Living

# Natural Solutions for Pain-Free Living

## LASTING RELIEF FOR FLEXIBLE JOINTS, STRONG BONES AND ACHE-FREE MUSCLES

### SHAWN M. TALBOTT, Ph.D.

*Author of* THE CORTISOL CONNECTION

& the Editors of SupplementWatch.com

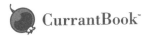 CurrantBook

Library of Congress Cataloging-in-Publication Data
Talbott, Shawn M.
Natural solutions for pain-free living : lasting relief for flexible joints, strong bones and ache-free muscles / Shawn Talbott, and the editors of Supplementwatch.com.
     p. cm.
Includes bibliographical references and index.
ISBN-13: 978-0-9711407-4-5 (alk. paper)
1. Chronic pain--Treatment. 2. Connective tissues--Diseases--Treatment. 3. Joints--Diseases--Treatment. 4. Dietary supplements. I. Title.
RB127.T35 2006
616'.0472--dc22

                                    2006001806

For ordering or other information, please contact:
Currant Book
311 East 100 North
Springville, Utah 84663
(801) 489-5576
info@currantbook.com
www.currantbook.com

Printed in the United States of America

## Dedication

This book is dedicated to my partner in business and in life—my lovely wife Julie. I could not be more grateful for her intelligence, thoughtful feedback, and enduring support while I wrote this book. And to our two wonderful kids, Alexander and Courtney, who both do their best to keep me young and flexible.

## Acknowledgments

Many thanks to Chef Michael Saccone for the excellent (and delicious) recipes that he provided. Each of these outstanding meals was created with ingredients to naturally control tissue inflammation and cellular oxidation, two of the most damaging biochemical processes in the body. Chef Saccone has succeeded in crafting a range of delectable recipes that not only taste great, but are good for you as well.

# Contents

# Author's Note

More than half of increased health care costs over the last ten years are the result of the increasing costs of pharmaceutical drugs—and yet complications from their use are the fourth leading cause of disease. Nowhere do we see the combination of high costs with extreme and dangerous side effects so dramatically as with the example of the COX-2-inhibitor class of arthritis drugs. These drugs have been taken by millions of Americans—and they've killed thousands (from increased incidence of heart attacks and strokes)—while simultaneously generating billions of dollars in profits for multinational drug companies.

Isn't there a better way? Of course there is, and we've known about many of these natural options for thousands of years. One of the most fascinating aspects of natural treatment options is finding new ways in which ancient remedies can help alleviate suffering from modern diseases. I have devoted my career as a nutritional biochemist to the discovery and development of natural options for promoting a healthy lifestyle. My ongoing mantra during this time—as it is today—has been to use the science of today plus the wisdom and tradition of nature to create the health of the future.

Among adults, nearly 10 percent of those who use NSAID drugs (non-steroidal anti-inflammatory drugs such as ibuprofen) will require hospitalization due to serious gastrointestinal toxicity (such as ulcers and stomach bleeding). In a 1998 study in the *American Journal of Medicine,* researchers reported that more than 107,000 people are admitted each year to hospitals—and another 17,000 die each year—as a direct result of complications due to the use of NSAIDs. This is a problem.

Toward the end of 1998, the Food and Drug Administration approved the drug we know as Celebrex (celecoxib) to treat arthritis pain. In its first nine months on the market, Celebrex racked up more than $1 billion in sales. The drug company Merck introduced its own COX-2 drug (Vioxx) a few months later and generated about the same $1 billion in sales in about half the time as Celebrex. Now, more than seven years later, we know that these COX-2 drugs weren't the miracle we were promised. In fact, now that the drug companies have been forced to give up their hidden files, we know that these drugs are no more effective at relieving pain than the aspirin in your medicine cabinet—and we also know that they're killing thousands of us (by causing heart attacks and stroke).

Should you be outraged? Absolutely! Should you look for alternatives to the expensive synthetic drugs that are being pushed on you to cure one disease while causing many others? Of course—and that's what I hope this book can do for you.

# 1

PAIN-FREE LIVING:
UNDERSTANDING INFLAMMATORY
BALANCE

Right now, there are approximately 30 million Americans with osteoporosis, 50 million with arthritis, and well over 100 million who suffer a sports-related injury each year. Overall, about one-eighth of the U.S. population suffers from some type of chronic pain—and about 80 percent of the adult population will suffer from back pain at some point in their lives. Back pain is the third most common reason for a visit to the doctor and the leading cause of activity limitation in adults under the age of fifty.

As the U.S. population ages, the total number of people with disability or functional impairment related to their bones and joints is expected to skyrocket. At this writing, more than 70 percent of the elderly suffer from some form of osteoarthritis of the knee joint. Over the next one to twenty years, an estimated 250 million people will be affected by joint and bone issues, and millions more will lose some degree of flexibility and mobility to other connective tissue ailments. Sobering statistics to be sure, but when considered in light of the dramatic increase in active lifestyles and sports participation among older Americans (up nearly 60 percent since 1990), it is clear that many people are not quite ready to accept these inevitable consequences of aging as part of their future. Dramatic breakthroughs in nutritional biochemistry, exercise physiology, and sports medicine have begun to change the way health professionals, and the public at large, think about the treatment and prevention of these conditions.

*Natural Solutions for Pain-Free Living* shows you how maintaining normal inflammatory balance in the body can support connective tissue health and help reduce suffering from arthritis, osteoporosis, fibromyalgia, low-back pain, and a wide range of connective tissue ailments. Specifically, *Pain-Free Living* focuses on the benefits of including natural dietary supplements within a larger program of nutrition and exercise for joint flexibility, bone strength, and tissue repair. It is my aim to guide you, step-by-step, through the complicated process of discovering, developing, and designing your own individualized program for connective tissue health.

## Understanding Connective Tissue and Inflammatory Balance

Why do you hurt? You can think of pain and inflammation as different sides of a coin—front and back or heads and tails—whatever analogy you prefer. The point is that pain and inflammation are driven by different—but related—biochemical factors. The good news is that we have a number of natural options that are safe and effective for controlling both pain and inflammation.

Pain and inflammation are normal body processes; without them we would literally not be able to survive for very long. Pain is a signal to your body that damage is occurring and you need to stop doing whatever is causing that damage.

Inflammation is a process controlled by the immune system that protects us from invading bacteria and viruses, but also helps regulate heart function, blood flow, and many vital functions. Keeping a normal balance of pain signals and inflammatory balance is vital to good health and well-being. When this balance becomes disrupted—or unbalanced—we experience more inflammation and pain and less flexibility and mobility. When we have too much inflammation, this process that is supposed to be protecting us actually causes more and more damage. For example, an overactive inflammatory response is known to stimulate bone breakdown (leading to osteoporosis) and interfere with cartilage repair (leading to a worsening of arthritis). Inflammation is also involved in emotional balance and brain function—so when our bodies experience too much inflammation, we simply don't feel happy and we feel mentally exhausted.

Your doctor may have given your unbalanced inflammation another kind of label—one that ends in "-itis" (in medical terminology, the suffix "-itis" is used to denote inflammation). So you may have arthritis (inflammation of the joint—*arthros* is Latin for joint), or tendonitis (inflammation of the tendon), or fasciitis (inflammation of the fascia, the tough layer of connective tissue over muscles, tendons and ligaments that can become inflamed following excessive exercise, low-back pain, and fibromyalgia).

## NORMAL INFLAMMATORY BALANCE VERSUS CHRONIC INFLAMMATION

Your normal process of inflammation helps to dismantle and recycle older cartilage and other connective tissues that have become damaged, worn-out or simply need repairing.

This process is called turnover—where older tissue is replaced with newer tissue. When we're young (before the age of thirty or so) this turnover process is perfectly balanced—for every bit of cartilage that is damaged and removed—another similar (or greater) bit is put in its place. This means that, under normal circumstances, we're always making our connective tissue—our cartilage and bones and muscles and tendons and ligaments—stronger and more resilient. After about age thirty, however, our turnover process becomes a bit less efficient year after year. This causes a very slight loss of healthy tissue—where we break down and remove a certain amount, but the amount of healthy tissue added back is just a little bit less than it should be. As we age, the turnover process becomes less and less efficient and our body's ability to heal itself from injury is reduced. This imbalance in tissue turnover and inflammatory balance is the primary cause of the loss of flexibility and the various "-itis" diseases that we all tend to encounter as we age.

These normal repair mechanisms start to dwindle as we age, and, ironically, the very inflammatory process that has been helping us to turn over older tissue into healthy new tissue can completely turn on us—leading to problems with pain, mobility, and flexibility. The very same inflammatory process that naturally governs our body's repair and protection now starts to accelerate tissue breakdown and impede its repair. The end result, as you may have already experienced, is that our tissues literally begin to fall apart. Cartilage degrades, muscles lose tone, ligaments and tendons creak, and bones become brittle.

Let's keep in mind that not all inflammation is bad—remember that inflammation is part of the normal healing and turnover process for any tissue. It's just when we get too much inflammation that things go awry. When this happens, healing is suppressed and tissue destruction is accelerated—your body simply cannot heal itself or stop the damage when the inflammatory process is unbalanced. To illustrate this point, think about the ocean crashing against a protective seawall. The seawall is your joint and other tissues, and the ocean is your inflammatory process. Over time, that wall will become broken and weakened by the crashing waves and will need to be repaired back to optimal function. If the pace of repair fails to keep up with the pace of destruction, then the seawall fails and the ocean comes rushing in (leading to total destruction and dysfunction). We need to maintain the integrity of the seawall (your joint) by keeping up with repair and maintenance, but we can't even do that if the ocean is continually crashing down on us.

Luckily, there is a plethora of scientific and medical evidence that shows us how to use diet, exercise, and supplementation to calm the ocean (to reduce damage caused by excessive inflammation) and accelerate tissue repair (keep that seawall intact). It's all a question of balance. We want to maintain that normal inflammatory balance so we can maintain a normal pace of tissue turnover, and thus balance healthy tissue, flexibility, and mobility. As soon as we fall out of inflammatory balance—even by a little bit—we see a little bit more tissue deterioration, leading to a little more inflammation and still more tissue breakdown. Once this vicious cycle of inflammation/damage has begun, it can be very difficult to stop—unless you have a comprehensive plan to rebalance inflammation from multiple perspectives.

# The Biochemistry of Inflammation

Before we can begin to understand the limitations and dangers of synthetic drugs—and why the many options for natural modifiers of pain and inflammation do not share the same side effects, we need a quick lesson about the biochemistry of inflammation. Much of your body's inflammatory response is regulated by two enzymes—one called cyclooxygenase (COX for short) and another called 5-lipoxygenase (5-LO for short). The COX enzyme can be further divided into COX-1 and COX-2, with COX-1 being the good form (because it protects our stomachs and kidneys) and COX-2 being the bad form of the enzyme (because it is the form responsible for creating prostaglandins, a group of inflammatory chemicals, as well as arachidonic acid, another inflammatory chemical). The COX-2 cousin enzyme, 5-LO, also uses arachidonic acid to create inflammatory chemicals—so it makes a lot of sense to control both COX-2 and 5-LO at the same time. There is also a related lipoxygenase enzyme called 12-LO that converts arachidonic acid into highly inflammatory compounds known as thromboxanes and eicosanoids. I'll outline some specific solutions for balancing the activity of all of these inflammatory enzymes with natural products in coming sections.

How many natural options would you guess are available for controlling COX-2 and 5-LO and 12-LO? Dozens! How many drugs can do all this? Zero! Why? Mostly because a multinational drug company can't make a billion dollars a year in profits by selling leaves, roots or plant extracts. Instead, they can synthesize their own "better" version of nature, patent it, and sell it at high profits with the blessing of the

Food and Drug Administration (FDA). Natural products, on the other hand, often work just as well (and in some cases better) as many synthetic drugs; they work in ways that the drugs can't; and they deliver benefits without the side effects that are all too common with the growing array of drugs entering the market each year.

In the early 1990s, the drug companies figured that if they could create a molecule that stopped just the COX-2 enzyme (leaving COX-1 alone), then they might be able to control pain and inflammation without the nasty side effects associated with drugs like ibuprofen (Advil), naproxen (Aleve), and aspirin (each of which can get rid of your headache, but also destroys your stomach lining and your kidneys because they all interfere with both COX-1 and COX-2). The idea of creating a selective COX-2 inhibitor was a good one ("on paper" as they say)—except for the fact that after drug companies learned these drugs were causing heart attacks and strokes, they insisted on continuing to sell them at huge profits. More on this later.

As drug companies will often do, they looked first to nature to see if any plants, herbs, or other natural products contained any clues to inhibition of the COX enzyme. Lo and behold! They found hundreds of plants with powerful anti-inflammatory and pain-controlling effects—some via the COX enzymes, some via the 5-LO enzyme, and even others through completely novel biochemical mechanisms. Also, as drug companies will always do, they took this knowledge and turned their back on nature—arrogantly believing that they could do better by synthetically creating a new-to-the-world molecule that more powerfully interfered with the inflammatory enzymes. The result was two drugs: Celebrex, which inhibits COX-2 about 400 times more powerfully than it does COX-1; and Vioxx, which inhibits COX-2 about 1,000 times more powerfully than COX-1. Both of these drugs are marvels of synthetic chemical engineering—but they are also prime examples of science run amok in the pursuit of profits. You've probably heard your mother say something like, "You'd cut off your own nose to spite your face," when you were being unreasonable as a child—well, the COX-2 class of drugs was exactly the same scenario—with drug companies encouraging you to gulp drugs that controlled your achy knee but destroyed your heart and blood vessels. It's a sad state of affairs when average Americans are being told that they only have two choices for controlling pain—take the older pain killers (NSAIDs) that temporarily relieve pain, but also wreck their stomachs—or take the newer painkillers (COX-2 inhibitors) that temporarily relieve pain, but damage their hearts. There are better options.

Okay, back to the biochemistry of inflammation. When a tissue is damaged—whether from infection or trauma or unbalanced turnover—it releases signaling chemicals called cytokines. These cytokines are like flare guns or a call for help that signal surrounding cells, as well as cells from the immune system, to jump into action to stop and repair the damage. One role of the cytokines is to call white blood cells into the area to help clean up the damaged tissue (the rushing blood leads to the recognizable redness, warmth, and swelling common to many injuries). As the white blood cells rush to the damaged area, they release more and more of their own inflammatory chemicals. This blast of inflammation is intended to cause even more tissue destruction as a way to either kill bacteria and viruses or take away damaged tissue and set the stage for repair efforts to begin. As you can imagine, this part of the inflammatory process is supposed to be short-term, and if it continued without shutting down, you'd simply continue to destroy your own tissue without ever rebuilding healthy tissue in its place. Unfortunately, this never-shut-down scenario precisely describes the chronic inflammation and constant state of tissue destruction under which millions of Americans live their lives every day. The solution, then, is to get the body out of its hyper-inflammatory state of destruction and back into a rebalanced state of repair.

## Chronic Inflammation: The World on Fire

It may help you to think of chronic inflammation as you would think of a fire in an apartment building. Let's say you live in a twenty-story apartment building (your joint) and a fire (inflammation) breaks out on the fifteenth floor. The fire causes destruction (tissue damage) to the entire fifteenth floor, but your penthouse apartment on the twentieth floor is fine. To put out the fire, you call in the firefighters (white blood cells), which may cause a bit more damage by spraying water and tearing down some walls—all in an effort to solve the bigger problem of putting out the fire. Let's now say that the fifteenth floor is a complete loss—while other floors suffer some repairable damage (water damage on the fourteenth floor and smoke damage on the sixteenth floor). The repair process begins on all three floors—carpenters, painters, and other builders are brought in to repair the damage. On fourteen and sixteen, where the damage is less severe, the repair process might be complete within a few weeks—while on fifteen where the fire was concentrated and the damage was most severe, the repair process may take a year.

Your body also has an entire team of builder cells in each

and every tissue—in cartilage they are called chondrocytes, in bone we call them osteoblasts, in muscles we know them as myocytes, in skin and some other tissues we have fibroblasts—the list goes on and on. In your own tissues, you can have the equivalent of a raging fire and firefighting (tissue damage and inflammation)—but if you're not able to shut off this process (that is, your inflammatory balance is thrown off by something), then your body is in a continual state of destruction and pain. You'll never be able to get to the rebuilding and repair stage unless you can shut off those chronic inflammatory signals.

## A Natural and Balanced Approach

If the inflammation process is a multifaceted chain reaction of biochemical events, then shouldn't your approach to controlling inflammation also be multifaceted? Of course it should! This is one of the many ways in which synthetic single-action pharmaceutical drugs fail miserably. Drugs work on one mechanism and they do it in a very powerful way—sometimes too powerfully (leading to serious side effects). If the recent history of medicine has taught us anything, it is that these modern single-action pharmaceutical drugs, these synthetic silver bullets previously unknown in nature, can have serious adverse consequences.

Popping a pill such as an aspirin or ibuprofen or one of the newer prescription drugs to control your pain is certainly not the answer. While these drugs may offer a short-term reduction in sensations of pain, they do nothing to address the root of the problem (restoring inflammatory balance). In fact, by strongly inhibiting the COX-2 enzyme and related inflammatory pathways such as prostaglandin production, these drugs can actually reduce tissue repair (especially for joint cartilage) and lead to severe damage in other tissues such as kidneys, liver, heart, and the entire gastrointestinal system (including gastric ulcers, stomach bleeding, and death).

The term COX-2 inhibitor generally refers to synthetic pharmaceutical drugs that interfere with the key enzyme involved with increasing inflammation and pain in the body. Many people have heard of the synthetic COX-2 drugs such as Vioxx, Bextra, and Celebrex (the first two have been forced off the market for causing heart attacks and the third is under investigation now for the same heart risks). However, very few people know that thousands of years ago, ancient herbal practitioners were prescribing all-natural herbal COX-2 inhibitors to control pain and inflammation. What these traditional healers did not know at the time, but what we know now, thanks to advances in nutritional biochemistry, is that these natural anti-inflammatory nutrients were simultaneously effective at controlling inflammation in many ways. This balanced approach is not only associated with a greater degree of overall effectiveness, but also with a restoration of normal tissue function and with fewer side effects. As is so often the case, however, the drug industry has tried to synthetically copy the extraordinary healing properties and powers of natural medicine—only to cause even more suffering and death. Luckily for us, those herbs and natural products cannot be owned by the drug companies—keeping them widely available for everyone to enjoy the benefits of controlling pain and inflammation—naturally, safely and effectively.

In the coming chapters, you will learn about the myriad natural options for naturally controlling pain and inflammation, improving mobility and flexibility, and actually rebuilding damaged tissues for long-term well-being. Before we turn our attention to the many solutions available to you, it is important to understand the current situation with the dangerous class of COX-2 drugs—what they are, how they work, and why they were allowed to remain on the market for so long after we learned that they were killing people.

## The COX-2 Catastrophe

In February 2005, the FDA convened an advisory meeting to look into the debacle surrounding the elevated risk of heart attack and stroke associated with the use of drugs in the COX-2 class of pain relievers. As mentioned earlier, this class of medications includes Merck's Vioxx (removed from the market), Pfizer's Celebrex (still on the market), and Bextra (pulled by Pfizer following the suggestion from the FDA to do so). All are under growing scrutiny for causing a variety of heart problems. In the near future, the FDA is expected to act on recommendations from its advisory committee to allow Vioxx back on the market (with a slim seventeen to fifteen vote in favor of allowing Merck to resume limited sales)— albeit with a stern black-box warning about the risk of heart problems (a black box is as tough as the FDA can generally get with already approved drugs). The FDA is not required to follow the recommendations of its advisory committee (but it usually does)—and with such a close vote and high stakes in terms of consumer health and litigation risk (which could rise as high as $50 billion by some estimates), the future of Vioxx is still very much up in the air. To defend itself against Vioxx claims, Merck has set aside a legal war chest of $675 million—an amount that might sound substantial, but pales in

Table 1. Pain Reliever Roulette

| DRUG | BRAND | OTC/RX | SALES (2003) | PROS | CONS |
|---|---|---|---|---|---|
| Acetaminophen | Tylenol | OTC | $760m | Reduces pain, easy on stomach | Does not reduce inflammation, may cause liver damage and lung damage, increases blood pressure |
| Aspirin | Bayer, Anacin | OTC | $240m | Reduces pain and inflammation, protects heart | Thins blood, can cause stomach ulcers, stokes, and kidney failure |
| Ibuprofen | Advil, Motrin | OTC | $680m | Reduces pain and inflammation, lower risk of stomach problems compared to aspirin | Ulcers and other gastrointestinal damage |
| Naproxen | Aleve | OTC | $250m | Reduces pain–especially in joints, long-lasting effect | Gastrointestinal damage, increased risk of heart attack and stroke |
| Rofecoxib | Vioxx | Rx | $1.8b | Reduces pain, easy on stomach | Doubles risk of heart attack and stroke |
| Celecoxib | Celebrex | Rx | $2.6b | Reduces pain, easy on stomach | Increased risk of heart attack /stroke |
| Valdecoxib | Bextra | Rx | $940m | Reduces pain | Gastrointestinal damage, increased risk of heart attack and stroke |
| Oxycodone | OxyContin | Rx | $1.9b | Reduces chronic pain | Addictive narcotic, patients can develop tolerance |

comparison to the $21.1 billion that Wyeth has paid to settle claims against the fen-phen weight loss drug, and the $1.11 billion that Bayer has paid (since February) on claims against its dangerous cholesterol drug Baycol. With 20 million people having taken Vioxx at some time since its launch in 1999, the legal costs for Merck could be huge.

To make matters even worse (giving you a headache if you didn't already have one) is the news that naproxen (the drug you may know as Aleve) and indeed the whole class of drugs in the category of NSAIDs (non-steroidal anti-inflammatory drugs) have also been implicated in a variety of adverse side effects from heart problems to gastrointestinal and liver problems (see Table 1). In addition, the pain killer acetaminophen (Tylenol), which is not strictly in the same chemical class as the other NSAIDs, has recently been linked to lung problems (associated with reduced levels of glutathione, an antioxidant) and high blood pressure. It seems that using synthetic drugs to control pain and inflammation is risky business no matter which drug you choose.

## COX-2 Inhibitors: The "Miracle" That Wasn't

Why are COX-2 drugs different from other painkillers? Aspirin and older painkillers like ibuprofen block both the COX-1 and COX-2 enzymes that are involved in pain and inflammation (COX-2), but which are also involved in normal function of the stomach, kidneys, and other tissues (COX-1). Vioxx, Celebrex, and Bextra are unique because they only block the COX-2 enzyme (a good and bad situation). Blocking COX-1 can reduce pain and actually improve heart health—but it also leads to gastrointestinal problems such as stomach ulcers (bad—it causes about 17,000 deaths—deaths!—each year from GI hemorrhaging induced by drugs like naproxen and ibuprofen). If a dietary supplement or herbal extract caused 17,000 deaths per year—or ever, you could bet that there would no longer be a natural products industry. But with drugs, this is apparently an acceptable outcome. The thought was that by leaving COX-1 alone and only blocking COX-2, you could get pain relief (in arthritic joints, for example) without the gut damage. This is indeed a boon for those chronic pain patients who do not find adequate relief from arthritis and other conditions with the older pain relievers. However, clinical trials have not shown Vioxx, Celebrex, or Bextra to be any more effective in managing pain than the older and cheaper painkillers—though there can be differences between patients where one drug may work better than another.

While I am in full support of the rights of patients and physicians to assess their own risk/benefit tolerance when it comes to drug choices and other self-care decisions, newer evidence is suggesting that both consumers and doctors may have not been given all of the information on which to base their decisions about COX-2 inhibiting drugs. For example, not only do COX-2 inhibitors not do anything for COX-1 (good for your gut and your aching knee, but bad for your heart), they may also suppress the formation of certain proteins that are needed to control blood clotting (thus increasing risk of heart problems). On this issue, I mostly agree with the FDA panel—that this class of drugs should be prescribed only to the very small group of patients who can draw enough unique pain/GI benefits to outweigh the increased risks to heart health—and not to the millions of consumers who were duped into believing that these "wonder" drugs were perfectly safe. I'm not alone in this regard—there are many medical experts who felt back in 1999 that the COX-2 inhibitor drugs simply did not offer an appreciable benefit-to-risk ratio, and thus should not have been approved (or perhaps should have been approved only for those arthritis patients at highest risk for ulcers and other GI problems).

## SLAUGHTERING THE COX-2 CASH COW

No sense looking back, however, because these drugs were approved and quickly became top sellers. From 1999 to 2003, Pfizer spent $406.3 million to market Celebrex ($114 million in 2004 alone), while Merck spent $459.8 million to market Vioxx ($81 million in 2004 alone)—and these numbers reflect only the direct-to-consumer ad spending (before Vioxx was pulled and the FDA asked Pfizer to stop marketing Celebrex). Pfizer bought Pharmacia in 2004 for an astounding $60 billion, largely because of Celebrex (which has become a $2.3 billion annual blockbuster for Pfizer and has been taken by about 28 million people worldwide). Bextra, another of Pfizer's COX-2 pain killers generates another $1 billion annually. Pfizer announced in December 2004 that it had agreed with the FDA to suspend all television, newspaper, and radio advertising of Celebrex to consumers (and modify ads to physicians). Vioxx was generating more than $2.5 billion in annual sales for Merck—partly based on direct-to-consumer advertising ($79 million in 2003 and $45 million in the first half of 2004). Its removal from the market in September 2004 resulted in a loss of nearly $28 billion in Merck's market capitalization—and liability estimates for the numerous lawsuits related to Vioxx's side effects may reach $50 billion. Ouch!

A large part of the growth in COX-2 drug sales is directly related to the direct advertising of prescription drugs to consumers—known as direct-to-consumer (DTC) ads, which exploded in 1997 when the FDA relaxed the rules governing what pharmaceutical companies could say about their drugs (and how they could say it). DTC advertising of prescription drugs rose 27 percent in 2004 to $4.44 billion, leading to widespread confusion on the part of consumers regarding the safety, risks, and side effects of drugs advertised during prime time. In a 2002 FDA survey of physicians, only 5 percent reported that their patients understood the risks of drugs appearing in DTC ads—and 59 percent of physicians reported that patients had asked for a drug by its brand name (resulting in a 57 percent rate of prescriptions written for that drug). Think about the efficiency of DTC advertising—consumers become "patients" when they are "informed" (or persuaded) about the drug through DTC advertising. Then, after demanding the drug by name, they usually get the advertised drug.

In the FDA advisory panel meeting in February 2005, several of the medical experts made a specific point to note that much of the existing DTC advertising minimizes the risks of the drugs and leads many patients to request and use those advertised drugs at an unnecessarily high rate. According to the latest data analysis, Merck's Vioxx (taken by more than 20 million people since its introduction in 1999) may have caused more than 140,000 heart attacks by the time it was taken off the market in September 2004. In a huge FDA analysis of data from 1.4 million patients taking Vioxx or other painkillers, those taking Vioxx over a five-year period had a 34 percent higher chance of coronary heart disease. Too bad the FDA didn't have this data in 1999 when they decided to unleash Vioxx on the American public or in 2002 when they decided only to force Merck to add a heart-risk warning to Vioxx labels (rather than remove the product from the market).

The current situation with the COX-2 drugs is not pretty. Several large studies published on the heart risks of Vioxx and Celebrex have shown a five-fold increase in heart attack risk from Vioxx (March 2000 study), a doubling of heart attack and stroke risk from Vioxx (September 2004 study), and a doubling of heart attack risk from Celebrex (December 2004 study), though Pfizer claims its own analysis of the data shows no problems (naturally).

It is important for consumers to understand that the risks of taking any prescription medication are always there (such as the doubling of heart risks with naproxen/Aleve suggested by an NIH study stopped in December 2005), but are often underappreciated by patients. The confusion is only compounded by the fact that in an American medical system that encourages physicians to push patients through HMOs every ten to fifteen minutes, there are not many doctors who can budget the twenty minutes needed to educate each patient about the pros and cons of the drugs or the many non-drug options that are available in the form of dietary supplements and other modalities. For example, I am simply astounded by the recent spate of drug ads informing consumers of the new "solution" to the dangers of COX-2 drugs—that being to combine their conventional painkillers (such as aspirin or naproxen, which cause GI bleeding) with drugs to reduce production of stomach acid (such as Pepcid or Prilosec). Does anybody else see a problem with this two-drugs-are-better-than-one "phaulty-pharma thinking"? The bottom line here is simply that there are no drugs with 100 percent safety, and it's looking more and more like a health gamble to take any drugs except in the most dire of circumstances.

## Natural Alternatives

The obvious challenge in selecting a natural option for pain relief is that you want something that is safe, natural, fast-acting, and long-lasting. It's a tall order to get all four wants in a single ingredient—but there are a growing number of products that offer a suitable range of options (mostly by combining the most effective ingredients into a single multi-faceted product solution).

One in six Americans lives in pain—with about 25 million Americans living with chronic low-back pain and close to 40 million more dealing with arthritis of the hands, knees, hips, and other joints. Getting rid of that pain is obviously an important consideration—especially if you're the one with the pain—but natural options found in dietary supplements should also be viewed not just as simple pain relievers, but also as agents to enhance the body's healing response.

Most of the OTC (over-the-counter) analgesics (painkillers) and non-steroidal anti-inflammatory drugs (NSAIDs) are safe and effective for short-term usage (two to three days at a time). NSAIDs do a great job of beating back the pounding from that headache, but they don't do a thing to help promote healing of your aching knee (in fact, in some important ways, these drugs may actually inhibit tissue healing, especially in the case of cartilage repair). There is also little doubt that NSAID therapy can lead to gastroduodenal ulcers—primarily due to their inhibition of prostaglandin production in the mucosal lining of the gastrointestinal tract (no mucus = no protection of stomach/intestinal lining = you digest yourself).

One of the most commonly used OTC drugs is aspirin. Often recommended for treating the pain of osteoarthritis, aspirin does a good job of relieving pain and inflammation. It's cheap, and when used regularly at a low dose, it can even help to prevent heart attacks and strokes. Unfortunately, for the pain of osteoarthritis, aspirin often must be used at a very high multi-gram dose, which invariably leads to gastric problems. This unfortunate choice—the pain in your joints or the ulcer in your belly—led to the introduction of the powerful COX-2 inhibitors such as Vioxx and Celebrex with promises of pain relief (though no better than drugs already available), and gastrointestinal protection (better than existing drugs, but only clearly better for Celebrex), and overall safety (clearly not the case, especially for your risk of heart disease and stroke).

Let's be clear about something before we start talking about any herbs of other supplements. Not all types of pain can be adequately addressed by natural medicines and dietary supplements, and in most cases of acute pain, you are probably better off using an OTC analgesic for a few days—but no more than that. When it comes to longer-term management of chronic pain and inflammation, it is indeed possible for consumers to use natural products combined with diet and exercise to manage their pain and stiffness—and also to reduce their dependency on drugs while also promoting tissue healing.

Such a regimen would ideally involve several aspects of using healing nutrients along with a regimen of proper diet, exercise, stretching, and stress management. Among the most popular nutritional supplements found in pain relief and arthritis-oriented products are glucosamine, chondroitin, MSM, HCP, proteolytic enzymes, papain, bromelain, devil's claw, boswellia, cetyl-myristeolate, fish oil, scutellaria, hyaluronic acid, type II collagen, white willow bark, and many others. As with most ingredients on the supplement scene, some are more effective than others—and some are particularly effective in specific cases.

## JOINT PAIN

When it comes to joint pain—particularly that associated with osteoarthritis and especially when in the knee, the first-line choice should be glucosamine. The downside, of course, is that glucosamine-based products typically take weeks to months to achieve therapeutic effect—meaning that you need to take them on faith for a period of time before noticing any reduction in pain or stiffness.

There are a number of new products hitting the market that provide a faster-acting form of pain relief added to the slower-acting joint rebuilders like glucosamine. Notable among these new additions to the marketplace is the herbal combination of scutellaria and acacia—a blend with good data showing analgesic and anti-inflammatory action leading to reduced pain in a matter of days/weeks versus weeks/months for most existing remedies. The combination of a faster-acting (though not immediate) herbal pain reliever with a slower-acting tissue builder such as glucosamine or hyaluronic acid is quite logical and I generally like to see products that build on this matrix approach (versus the single magical ingredient approach, which tends to fail on many fronts).

## MUSCLE AND SOFT TISSUE PAIN

If you have pain that migrates outside of the joint space (cartilage damage) to the muscles, tendons, ligaments, and other connective tissues, then your first-line choice is likely to be an anti-inflammatory herbal extract—such as boswellia, turmeric, ginger, avocado/soy extracts (ASUs), or the aforementioned scutellaria.

In terms of anti-inflammatory oils, the plain old fish oil that you may already be taking for your heart health is also a safe option for controlling inflammation (which may or may not work very well depending on the dose and the strength of the fish oil you choose). A more effective approach may be found in a specialized fatty acid blend known as cetyl myristeolate (CM). CM has been the subject of a handful of clinical studies showing reduced pain in arthritis (over 30–60 days) and following muscle injury.

The old standby for post-surgical wound healing and for most soft-tissue sports injuries is a blend of proteolytic enzymes. Numerous studies have shown a reduction in inflammation and an acceleration of wound healing with supplementation—and professional and recreational athletes the world over routinely reach for proteolytic enzyme preparations to help promote healing and recovery from minor soft tissue injuries. Other much-hyped ingredients such as MSM, willow bark, licorice, feverfew, and others should be viewed as support ingredients (won't hurt, might help) in formulations based upon the aforementioned effective ingredients.

## Choosing and Using

There are literally hundreds of choices among natural options for pain relief and tissue healing—and while many or most of these nutrients and herbal extracts may be perfectly suitable as added support ingredients within broadly formulated blends, your biggest bang for the buck will be found with combinations of nutrients that can deliver as many of the following benefits as possible:

1. *Control inflammation and balance the inflammatory cascade*
   a. Balance the COX-2 enzyme (Cyclo-Oxygenase-2)
   b. Balance the 5-LO enzyme (Lipo-Oxygenase)
   c. Restore inflammatory balance between inflammatory and anti-inflammatory cytokines/prostaglandins/thromboxanes/eicosanoids

2. *Control oxidation (which can lead to inflammation at the cellular level)*
   a. Include broad-spectrum antioxidants including natural vitamin E, vitamin C, flavonoids, carotenoids, and thiols

3. *Rebuild damaged tissues including all aspects of joint structure:*
   a. Cartilage
   b. Bones
   c. Muscles
   d. Tendons
   e. Ligaments

4. *Protect healthy tissues (from damage induced by inflammatory and oxidative compounds)*

In the forthcoming chapters, you'll learn about many of the most potent and balanced natural herbal supplements for controlling pain and inflammation and rebuilding/protecting tissues. Here is a brief overview of some of the most important:

### TURMERIC *(Curcuma longa)* AND GINGER *(Zingiber officinalis)*

Both turmeric and ginger are cousin herbs that have been used for centuries in the traditional Ayurvedic medicine of India and other parts of Asia. Ayurveda translates as "knowledge of life" and holds as a central concept that natural approaches to healing must be balanced to be most effective. Both herbs are termed in the Ayurvedic system as *vishwabhesaj*, translated as "universal medicines," because of their potent anti-inflammatory and antioxidant activities. Modern studies have shown that both turmeric and ginger can restore inflammatory balance through multiple mechanisms of action. For example, both of these spice herbs are known to modulate the metabolism of arachidonic acid (one of the pro-inflammatory products of omega-6 fatty acids), and reduce activity of the COX-2 and 5-LO enzymes. Ginger and turmeric also reduce the activity of another inflammatory enzyme known as 12-LO (12-lipoxygenase) that also metabolizes arachidonic acid. In doing so (inhibiting 12-LO), ginger and turmeric can inhibit the formation of other prostaglandins that can sensitize pain receptors—so a reduction in these inflammatory compounds leads to a direct reduction in both the causation and the perception of pain.

### SCUTELLARIA *(Scutellaria baicalensis)*

Scutellaria is also known as Baikal skullcap and is native to China, Korea, Japan, and parts of Russia. The root extract has been used for centuries in traditional Chinese medicine (TCM) as both an anti-inflammatory and promoter of wound healing. In these ancient systems of medicine, natural extracts were viewed as modulators of normal function—where they could help the body restore its own natural balance—rather than as cures in today's synthetic pharma-model. It is interesting to note that scutellaria is both a source of antioxidant flavonoids (which reduce COX-2 and 5-LO enzyme activity as well as help repair and protect tissues from damage) and melatonin (which reduces 12-LO activity). Melatonin is a naturally occurring hormone produced in the brain and has relaxation, calming, and mood-boosting effects. Melatonin supplementation can help promote restful sleep and because of its chemical/structural similarity to serotonin, it can help to boost mood and feelings of well-being. You might also be interested to know that melatonin also shares a structural relationship to indomethacin—a widely used painkiller in Europe and Japan. With all of this going for it, it's no wonder that scutellaria extract has been used in traditional medicine for controlling inflammation and pain, but also for controlling stress and boosting mood and mental outlook.

## BOSWELLIA (*Boswellia serrata*)

Boswellia is a traditional Indian herb used for centuries in Ayurvedic medicine for treating pain and inflammation. You might know boswellia by its more famous name of frankincense—which was given as one of the three valuable gifts (the others being gold and myrrh) to the baby Jesus by the three wise men in the biblical story (the wise men were Zoroastrian priests from Persia who, in those times, were charged with providing and communicating health and healing). Boswellia plants are a source of specific organic acid compounds that inhibit both COX-2 and 5-LO, as well as reduce the activity of a metalloprotein that degrades joint cartilage. This makes boswellia extract a single plant product that reduces inflammation and pain by at least three complementary mechanisms simultaneously.

### GRAPE SEED EXTRACT (*Vitis vinifera*)

The seed of the grape is one of the richest natural sources of a group of compounds known as polyphenols and as proanthocyanins—both of which are powerful antioxidants that may help slow the onset and spread of arthritis. Osteoarthritis, as you already know, is caused by a breakdown in the cartilage tissue of the joint—but it can be exacerbated and cartilage destruction can accelerate if the inflammatory process runs out of control. The polyphenol compounds in grape seed extract (and certain other plant extracts such as green tea and pine bark) are known to not only reduce the activity of the COX-2 enzyme (thus reducing inflammation), but also to help promote healing of the damaged tissue and protection of the newly formed healthy tissue from future damage.

## The Broad-Spectrum Dream Team

To reemphasize an important point—keep in mind that your inflammation and pain are not caused by any single aspect of biochemistry, but rather by by several aspects. It makes sense, then, to combat that pain by using multiple approaches—by modulating and restoring inflammatory balance using as many tools as you have access to. You might start with scutellaria or turmeric (each of which have hundreds of naturally occurring and biologically active compounds). But why not also incorporate other complementary natural products to fully address every aspect of the inflammatory cascade, tissue repair process, and ongoing protection of healthy tissues?

The overall effect of this combined approach is a restoration of inflammatory balance and a reduction in pain—but these overall effects come through several complementary mechanisms simultaneously. Think about how this is the exact opposite of how Vioxx or Celebrex or other synthetic drugs accomplish their effects (and side effects). These drugs are single synthetic molecules chemically engineered to do one thing (interfere with normal metabolism), while natural extracts like ginger, turmeric, grape seed, scutellaria, and many others have hundreds of naturally occurring compounds that work in a complementary fashion to rebalance an out-of-control inflammatory cascade.

Not only does this combinatorial matrix approach to supporting health make more sense, it's also more effective and safer in the long run. Not only do you have multiple mechanisms of action working simultaneously, but you have complementary and synergistic effects that actually help each ingredient work better in concert than it would on its own. It's the difference between listening to one person banging loudly on a bongo versus listening to a beautifully choreographed symphony played by a full orchestra. The recipes that follow in Chapter 7 will help you to incorporate a full orchestra of anti-inflammatory and antioxidant foods into your diet, and the dietary supplement recommendations throughout each chapter (and especially Chapter 5) will help you draft your own "dream team" of natural ingredients to restore your own normal inflammatory balance.

# 2

---

## CONNECTIVE TISSUE:
## THE FOUNDATION ON WHICH
## WE'RE BUILT

Now that you know something about the inflammatory process and why it's so important to maintain normal inflammatory balance, let's turn our attention to the specific tissues in your body that can benefit from restoring and maintaining this balance.

Before we get into an explanation about the ins and outs of my program—which I call the FlexCare Program—or how it can help you develop flexible joints, strong bones, and ache-free muscles for life (as the subtitle of this book promises), let's begin with the basics.

What is connective tissue? The term *connective tissue* describes a wide range of tissues in the body that collectively have an extracellular matrix that serves to support and protect organs. There are four basic types of connective tissue:

*Cartilage.* Found mostly in joints (between bones) with an extracellular matrix composed primarily of the tough fibrous protein called collagen (more about collagen later). Cartilage tissue is formed and maintained by specialized cells called chondrocytes. Inflammation within the joint space can accelerate the destruction of cartilage tissue and destroy healthy chrondrocytes.

*Bone.* Contains specialized bone-building cells called osteoblasts and bone-destroying cells called osteoclasts embedded in a mineralized extracellular matrix (collagen filled in with calcium, magnesium, boron, silicon, and other minerals). Bone obviously functions to provide support for the entire body, but when inflammation becomes chronic, bone tissue breaks down faster (due to increased osteoclast activity) and bone building and bone strength suffer (because osteoblast function is inhibited). Too much inflammation eventually leads to osteoporosis.

*Fibrous Connective Tissue.* The catch-all term that we apply to connective tissues such as ligaments, tendons, a portion of the muscles, and the fascia (a dense connective tissue covering over muscles that becomes chronically inflamed in fibromyalgia). These fibrous connective tissues help us get from point A to point B, but when they become inflamed, even the most basic activities become a painful ordeal.

*Blood/Circulatory System.* Functions in the transport of nutrients, oxygen, hormones, and numerous good and bad substances throughout the body. Its extracellular matrix of blood plasma and blood vessels has its main cellular component of red and white blood cells, as well as the fibroblasts that make up the structure of the vessels. Even though you might not think of your blood as becoming inflamed, we need to keep in mind that inflammation in one part of the body (your knee joint, for example) can travel via the blood to other parts of the body. So, the chronic inflammation of arthritis in your joint cartilage can lead to faster bone breakdown (inflammation in the bones), increased feelings of stiffness (inflammation in the fascia), a higher incidence of heart disease (inflammation in the blood vessels), an increased rate of depression (inflammation in the brain)—the list goes on and on with inflammation affecting each and every body system.

## Connective Tissue Turnover

Connective tissue is continually undergoing a process of breakdown and repair. This cycle of tearing down and building back up again is referred to as turnover and is a perfectly normal part of keeping all tissues at peak health. The turnover process allows connective tissues to adapt to stress and repair themselves after suffering damage. For instance, let's say you overdo it at the company softball game and wake up with stiff, achy muscles and joints the next morning. The pain and discomfort that you are feeling is a result of damage to your muscles, tendons, and ligaments caused by the stress and inflammation of overexertion. You already know that the pain and stiffness will eventually go away over the next couple of days—that's because your natural turnover process will begin to remove the damaged tissue and replace it with brand-new healthy tissue that is just a little bit stronger than it was before.

The connective tissue turnover process in all of your tissues can be influenced by a variety of factors including age, physical health, and nutrient intake. It doesn't take a rocket scientist to point out the wrinkling of skin, the stiffening of joints, and the graying (or loss) of hair as we age. We've known for decades that regular physical activity and proper nutrition can help delay or reverse some of the deterioration of our bodies. In fact, many of the losses in function considered to be inevitable consequences of aging are little more than minor inefficiencies and subtle deficits in this turnover process that have built up over many years.

For example, joint stiffness is probably the first consequence of aging that we notice. Why? Because we try to get up from the chair or carry something across the yard and we say, "Whoa, I never felt that before." What you're feeling in this situation is the result of years and years of accumulated stress (and inadequate repair) in your connective tissue. The very same process is at work throughout your body, from joints and bones, to muscles, tendons, and ligaments—and the key to maintaining optimal tissue function is to support and promote the naturally balanced turnover process.

Virtually each and every situation that we associate with aging can be directly attributed to the lifetime balance of degradation and repair within each tissue. In the innumerable cases that make us feel older (joint pain, weak muscles, stiff tendons and ligaments) a significant underlying relationship to connective tissue health exists. In each case, the balance between breakdown and repair has tilted in favor of connective tissue loss.

Even if tissue breakdown outpaces repair by just a very slight amount, the combined effect over the years will lead to dysfunction. If you could just give the balance a little bump—and either nudge the synthesis of connective tissue a little higher or push the breakdown of connective tissue a little lower—then you'd be back in balance. Even better, if you could stack the deck in your favor, by increasing connective tissue synthesis above the breakdown rate, then you could actually make gains in those areas that previously gave you grief. That's what the FlexCare Program in Chapter 6 can help you do—tilt the balance of connective tissue breakdown and repair back to your favor by controlling inflammation, oxidation, and tissue repair and protection (the key regulators of connective tissue metabolism).

## Connective Tissue Maintenance: Synthesis, Breakdown, and Repair

The process of connective tissue synthesis and repair is a complex chain of events involving the structural protein called collagen. Collagen synthesis begins deep within individual cells in each tissue. Amino acids are transported into the cell and added to the growing collagen chain—sort of like adding beads to a necklace. As the beads (amino acids) are added, the necklace (collagen molecule) gets longer. When three collagen molecules are finished, they are twisted together by a specialized group of enzymes to form a braided rope-like structure called a triple helix. This triple helix is then transported out of the cell for further processing. Once outside the cell, various reactions, some requiring enzymes and some occurring on their own with time, help bring these triple helix collagen molecules into the proper arrangement (amino acids => collagen molecules => triple helix => collagen fibrils => collagen fibers). Depending on the tissue involved, the collagen molecules may be arranged in fibers placed very close together (as in bone) or spaced a little farther apart (as in joint cartilage). The precise arrangement of each collagen fiber will help determine its ultimate function.

After the collagen fibers are in place, the real work has just begun—now you've got to maintain this complex collagen fiber arrangement against the repetitive strain of everyday events. To help maintain its strength and resiliency, collagen is continually undergoing a process of breakdown and rebuilding. This turnover process is really a recycling process that helps get rid of older collagen fibers that may be damaged or weakened, and replaces them with newer, healthier fibers that are stronger and more able to withstand strain. Just as public works crews are sent out to repair potholes in roads, your body has to fight an ongoing struggle to constantly maintain collagen and repair the connective tissue network.

Without this ongoing renewal and repair process of connective tissue turnover, small bits of daily damage would build up and result in a serious deterioration of the tissue. In joints, this might lead to painful arthritis; in bones, it might lead to a stress fracture or osteoporosis; and in muscles and tendons, the risk for strains, tears and back pain might be increased. These are the more serious potential risks, but there are a number of other adverse effects from an inadequate or inefficient connective tissue turnover process, such as premature wrinkling of skin and graying (or loss) of hair—even premature tooth loss.

## Connective Tissue and Aging

I certainly don't need to tell anybody reading this book that skin wrinkles as we age. Wrinkled skin is almost something that we've all come to accept as an inevitable part of the aging process. Have you ever stopped to wonder, though, just why it is that our skin wrinkles as we age? How about the fact that some people have more wrinkles than others? How about whether or not something can be done about it?

Well, there are a number of approaches that can be taken to help combat the appearance of wrinkles in the skin. Even more important, however, is to understand that by looking at our wrinkling skin, we can get a good idea about what is happening to the other connective tissues throughout your body. Even though you can't see your joint cartilage becoming "wrinkled" and damaged by runaway inflammation, the very same destructive "wrinkling" process is at work in each of your connective tissues.

The basic underlying reason that our skin wrinkles and other connective tissues break down faster with age is because we dry out. As we age, our bodies actually lose moisture little by little—and the end result is that we all shrivel up a bit. The drying out process can be accelerated by environmental factors such as prolonged exposure to the sun and smoking (both sources of oxidation) or by prolonged exposure to inflammatory chemicals such as cytokines and eicosanoids. Luckily, however, this drying out process can be slowed somewhat by eating the right foods, following the right exercise regimen, and supplementing with the right herbs and nutrients (more about this later).

With age, a number of noticeable changes in connective tissue structures become apparent. Connective tissue fibers lose their elasticity—so we may become "droopy" in areas of our body that used to be firm. Connective tissue begins to lose its ability to hold water, so our skin dries out and becomes dysfunctional. With age, cartilage cells lose their ability to produce new collagen, so we lose cartilage thickness and our joints begin to ache. Bones become weaker over time as the rate of collagen and mineral breakdown exceeds our ability to replace losses with healthy tissue. As a result of all these small changes in connective tissue structures, we slowly begin to lose flexibility and mobility. The end result—which often goes unnoticed until it's too late—is that we can't get around like we used to when we were younger (when our ability to maintain connective tissue was better). If we could just balance the connective tissue turnover process, or better yet, tip the scales slightly in our favor—we could balance out the destruction and repair of our vital connective tissues and prevent (or delay) some of the conditions that we normally associate with aging.

The following sections give a brief overview of the unique role that connective tissue plays in some of the principal tissues in the body. As mentioned previously, the chapters that follow will go into much more detail about the specific recommendations and suggested exercise and nutritional support for each tissue system.

## Joints: The Weakest Link

Your poor joints—they've long been treated like the crazy uncle in the family. You always knew they were there, they often gave you a great deal of grief, and you hoped that they would just stop bothering you. Well, I'm sorry to be the one to tell you—but unless you do something about those joints you're going to be sorry. Here's why:

*Reason 1.* Joint cartilage has a slow metabolism.
*Reason 2.* Joint cartilage has no blood supply.
*Reason 3.* Cartilage cells cannot replicate.
*Reason 4.* Cartilage breaks down as we age.
*Reason 5.* Joints need proper nutrition.

Articular cartilage is the name for the specific kind of cartilage that makes up the joints and keeps the ends of bones from rubbing together. It is composed of three major com-

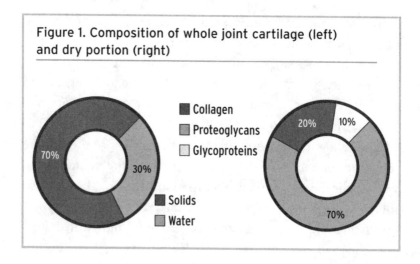

Figure 1. Composition of whole joint cartilage (left) and dry portion (right)

ponents: water for lubrication, collagen to provide structure, and proteoglycans to attract and hold water. Normal articular cartilage is about 70 percent water and 30 percent solids. Of the solid portion of cartilage, collagen accounts for about 70 percent, proteoglycans make up about 20 percent, and other proteins about 10 percent.

Cartilage is an interesting tissue. It has no blood supply and no nerve endings, yet it is very much alive. Joint cartilage is surrounded by a special kind of liquid called synovial fluid. The synovial fluid is vital to the health and function of joint cartilage. Without it, cartilage would die and we'd be in so much pain that we couldn't walk ten feet.

Because joint cartilage has no blood supply, the tissue must rely on the synovial fluid to deliver the nutrients that it needs to survive. Synovial fluid serves as the primary source of nutrition for the cartilage cells (chondrocytes). Nutrients such as amino acids, vitamins, and minerals are normally found in the circulation and are typically delivered to tissues through the blood vessels. In the case of cartilage, the nutrients have to first travel out of the blood, into the synovial fluid, and then into the cartilage tissue. This is a time-consuming delivery process, but it is one that we can speed up a bit by providing higher levels of specific nutrients in the diet and by encouraging nutrient transfer between tissues via exercise.

Specific nutrient recommendations for joint cartilage are presented in Chapters 5 and 6. In general, however, a higher blood level of a particular nutrient will result in a faster transfer of that nutrient into the synovial fluid and a more rapid delivery to the cartilage cells. The faster you can get the proper nutrients to the site of connective tissue production, the more quickly you can stimulate synthesis of healthy cartilage.

Regular physical activity is also an essential component of maintaining healthy joints because exercise causes a compression/relaxation effect on joint cartilage and helps to encourage the transfer of nutrients from the circulation into the synovial fluid and into the cartilage tissue. In fact, physical activity is so important, that any kind of prolonged inactivity or immobilization of any joint will result in cartilage degeneration.

## Bones: More Than Just Calcium

If you think that chewing a few Tums every day is going to protect you from osteoporosis, you had better think again. Contrary to popular belief, bones are a heck of a lot more than just calcium. Don't get me wrong—adequate calcium intake is certainly one of the most important factors in achieving and maintaining optimal bone strength. With fewer than 20 percent of Americans consuming enough calcium each day, many of us have come to accept the fact that we either have to take calcium supplements or we'll never get up to the daily recommended level—that's just fine. It is very important to understand, however, that strong, healthy bones need calcium to be balanced with magnesium, boron, and silicon, but also need vitamins C, D, and K to help those minerals to perform their bone-strengthening activities.

Minerals make up about 70 percent of the weight of bones (mostly calcium, phosphorous, and magnesium), with protein contributing about 20 percent, and water the remaining 10 percent. If we forget about the mineral portion for a minute and concentrate on the protein portion, we see that almost all (90 percent) of the protein in bone comes from collagen. Now consider the fact that this protein portion is what gives bones their toughness, durability, and resistance to bending. Without collagen, bones have no more strength than a stick of chalk. A bone made only of calcium would snap under the stress of standing and could never hold up to the strain of walking or running. The amazing strength of human bones is

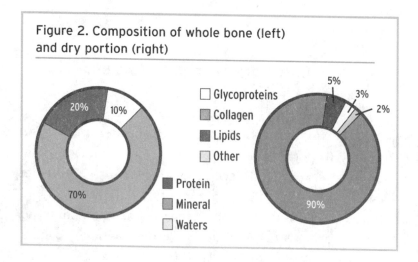

Figure 2. Composition of whole bone (left) and dry portion (right)

Glycoproteins
Collagen
Lipids
Other

Protein
Mineral
Waters

actually a bit better than the strength of steel (when compared on a pound-per-pound basis), and is due in large part to the unique composition of minerals, connective tissue, and water.

Maintaining an adequate amount of bone tissue becomes more and more important as we age—particularly for women. With age, there is a progressive loss of bone mass, which increases the risk of developing osteoporosis and fractures from weak bones. Exercise and dietary patterns have a lot to do with the achievement and maintenance of adequate bone mass—and the FlexCare Program outlined in Chapter 6 will do as much for your bones as it will for your joints and the rest of your body.

Adequate nutrition and regular exercise are extremely important for bone health. Aside from consuming enough calcium every day, a number of other vitamins, minerals, and non-nutrient food components can help increase bone density and strength. Exercise, particularly resistance training or weight lifting, is known to stimulate bone formation, enhance bone strength, and decrease the risk of osteoporosis. More specific diet and exercise recommendations for bone health can be found in Chapters 5 and 6.

## Muscles, Tendons and Ligaments: Getting from Here to There

Anybody who is physically active or involved in any kind of competitive or recreational sports should be concerned about proper muscle function. When most of us think about muscles, we automatically think about them in terms of size and strength and the amount of force they can generate. After all, it's our muscles that allow us to move around, to run, to jump, and to be active.

There is certainly no denying that one of our major concerns when it comes to exercise performance is the optimal combination of training and recovery to encourage muscles to grow bigger and stronger. Whether you consider yourself a serious athlete or more of a weekend warrior, the exercise that you do has a tremendous impact on the health of your connective tissue (in ways that are both good and bad). The positive effects of exercise are to stimulate bone formation, provide compression to joint cartilage, and strengthen muscle tissue. The detrimental side of excessive physical activity or exercise without adequate recovery can reveal itself as joint stiffness, stress fractures, and tendon or muscle strains.

The outer layer of tissue surrounding muscle fibers, called fascia, is almost 100 percent collagen and is responsible for helping to maintain the strength and functional integrity of the muscle fibers. If this fascia is disrupted or weakened, the end result is either a weak muscle with reduced ability to generate force or a muscle at higher risk for injury (or both). In a similar fashion, tendons, which are about 85 percent collagen fibers, need to remain strong and healthy in order to respond to the high forces generated by physical activity.

Unless you have ever suffered a tendon strain or a ligament sprain, you have probably not thought much about the health of these structures. Tendons are very dense, tough tissues that are responsible for connecting muscles to bone. Tendons allow us to make forceful muscle contractions during exercise. An example of a major tendon is the Achilles tendon, which attaches the calf muscle (gastrocnemius) to the heel of the foot and plays a major role during jumping and running.

Ligaments are also extremely dense and tough tissues, but

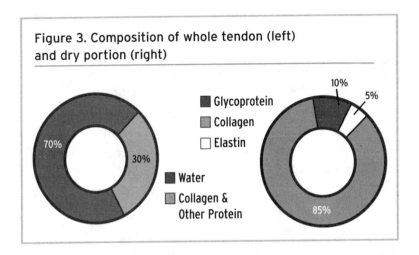

Figure 3. Composition of whole tendon (left) and dry portion (right)

their main function is to connect bone to bone. A major ligament in the body, the anterior cruciate ligament (or ACL), is needed to attach the upper leg bone (the femur) to the lower leg bone (the tibia) and provide support to the knee joint. An injury to the ACL, as in many sports injuries, often results in a loss of strength and stability in the knee joint. A great many professional athletes have been forced into early retirement by ACL injuries.

Tendons and ligaments are about 85 percent collagen fibers, with a small amount of special elastic protein fibers to provide some flexibility. Tendons and ligaments differ somewhat in their connective tissue fiber arrangements. In tendons, the connective tissue fibers are aligned in more of a side-by-side fashion (to allow more flexibility), while those in ligaments have more of a crisscross pattern (to provide less stretch and more support). In both cases, optimal connective tissue turnover is needed to repair accumulated damage so that remaining tissue can respond to the high forces generated by daily activity.

# My Own Story

I have to be perfectly honest with you here: I never even thought about ligaments as a part of the body that needed specific nutrition until a few years ago. It happened like this. I was out for my morning run, covering a route that I must have run over a hundred times before, when wham!—I stepped off a curb the wrong way and rolled my ankle all the way over to the pavement. I can't say that there was a whole lot of initial pain, just the feeling that my ankle was not a happy customer. The swelling—now that was another story. Within a matter of seconds, I looked like I was smuggling a grapefruit in my left sock—not a pretty picture. To make a long story short, the diagnosis was a third-degree sprain (torn ligament) that required crutches and sixteen weeks to heal. Even after more than four months of rest, ice, and physical therapy, the ligaments on that side of my ankle were weak. I felt as if my foot would just flop over to the side if I put any pressure on it.

My options at the time were to either wear an ankle brace or have surgery—otherwise I was destined to be plagued with this weak ankle forever (an "Achilles ankle," so to speak). My story is not much different from the thousands of people each year who injure their knee or ankle ligaments while downhill skiing or shooting hoops. The difference now, however, is that we know more about optimal nutrition and supplementation, we know more about how to tame the ongoing inflammatory process, and we know that we can combine the best parts of diet and exercise to accelerate healing.

# Summary

Now you know a little something about what connective tissue is and the important role that it plays in maintaining the structural integrity of the body. You have also been introduced to the general concept of harnessing the body's own metabolic machinery to support the process of connective tissue repair and renewal. In the coming chapters, you'll learn how aging can influence inflammatory balance and the process of connective tissue turnover. But you'll also learn how diet, exercise, and supplements can help turn metabolism in your favor to prevent tissue damage and actually restore mobility and flexibility throughout your entire body.

# 3

THE GRAYING OF AMERICA:
AGING AS A BALANCE
BETWEEN CONNECTIVE TISSUE
BREAKDOWN AND REPAIR

**M**uch of what we know as aging today is little more than an accumulation, over years and years, of deficits in connective tissue repair. The field of anti-aging research is still in its infancy (see how good it is!) and as such, some of the ideas that are often touted as miraculous fountain-of-youth remedies are a bit wacky. When it comes to the maintenance of connective tissue, however, we can substantiate these anti-aging effects and benefits with hard scientific data. By addressing the nutritional needs of this complex tissue, we can often slow or even reverse some of the consequences that many people view (incorrectly) as the inevitable effects of getting older.

One of the popular definitions of aging is, "the process of changing with time, especially during the later part of life." True enough, but what most of us understand as aging is more about creaking joints, stiff muscles, wrinkling skin, thinning hair, spreading waistlines, and diminishing energy levels. But it doesn't have to be this way. There are millions of people who get older (in terms of years on this planet), but don't look much older—and they certainly don't feel much older. These are the folks that we call the successful aging population, and this chapter reveals many of their secrets for maintaining their youthful appearance—but more importantly, their youthful connective tissue and the freedom of flexibility and mobility that results.

## Metabolic Aging

There are several approaches that can help accomplish this goal of successful aging. First, let's look at some of the causes of aging and the metabolic factors that contribute to the aging process. These factors are important for all of us to understand because in understanding them, we can better plan our attack against the aging process—and in doing so, look and feel better than ever.

There are four primary metabolic factors that contribute to what most of us understand as aging. Each of these areas of metabolism can lead to accelerated aging when unbalanced (in a negative direction), but can also lead to a dramatic anti-aging effect when balanced or temporarily unbalanced (in a positive direction). Also, and importantly, each of these four aspects of metabolism is intimately intertwined and interdependent on the others—a situation that can be good (if you can control all four simultaneously), but which can also be very frustrating (as in controlling one area, while another area continues to cause problems).

For example, scientists have known for decades that highly reactive oxygen molecules called free radicals are a primary source of aging because they cause damage (oxidation) to cellular structures (membranes, mitochondria, and DNA), leading to cellular dysfunction. Controlling free-radical metabolism would seem to be a viable anti-aging approach—and it is—up to a point. Unfortunately, another metabolic process, inflammation (caused by eicosanoids, cytokines, prostaglandins, and other molecules), can also accelerate cellular damage and aging—and even worse, oxidation can lead to inflammation and vice-versa. Adding to the confusion is the recent scientific understanding that inflammatory control is tightly linked to glucose levels in the blood—meaning that fluctuations in blood sugar (up or down) can lead to fluctuations in inflammatory balance and thus in free-radical load. Higher levels of glucose in the blood lead to glycation of proteins (attachment of sugar molecules to the protein), including collagen and related proteins in connective tissues. Glycated molecules tend to be dysfunctional—so connective tissues have reduced strength, break down faster, and lose much of their elasticity. As a result, skin sags and wrinkles, joints creak and pop, and muscles become stiff and inflexible. If all that weren't bad enough, we also know that stress, and the primary stress hormone cortisol, can lead to higher blood sugar levels (increasing glycation) and higher levels of inflammation (setting off a chain reaction between eicosanoids and free radicals), which leads to greater levels of oxidative damage to cells throughout the body—including connective tissue in joints, bones, muscles, tendons, and ligaments.

The FlexCare Program outlined later in the book modulates each and every one of these metabolic factors to fully address the overall aging process:

*Inflammation* is caused by inflammatory prostaglandins, eicosanoids, and cytokines. These are hormone-like compounds produced by cells to communicate with one another. The immune system is the primary source of eicosanoids—with both inflammatory and anti-inflammatory forms existing in the body at all times. The problem with eicosanoids is not that they are bad—but rather that having too many of the inflammatory type and too few of the anti-inflammatory type leads directly to tissue damage as well as to higher levels of both free radicals (and the oxidative damage they cause) and cortisol overexposure (leading to glycation and the resulting tissue damage).

Eicosanoids can be controlled by limiting your intake of inflammatory fatty acids (such as omega-6 fatty acids found in most vegetable oils) and increasing your intake of anti-inflammatory fatty acids (such as omega-3 fatty acids found in fatty fish and fish oil supplements). Omega-3 fatty acids can also control cortisol levels (see below). Spices such as turmeric and ginger can directly control both inflammatory eicosanoids as well as oxidative free radicals (see below).

*Oxidation* is caused by highly reactive oxygen molecules called free radicals that lead to damage of cellular membranes and DNA. Oxidized cells do not perform optimally and can lead to disease and dysfunction in all tissues, including connective tissues. Free radicals are directly associated with connective tissue damage and with elevated levels of inflammation, which leads to further tissue dysfunction.

Free radicals can be controlled by antioxidants such as vitamin C, vitamin E, alpha lipoic acid, flavonoids (as in grape seed, green tea, citrus, and others), and carotenoids (such as beta-carotene, lycopene, lutein, and others). Antioxidants can be found in brightly colored fruits and vegetables as well as in dietary supplements.

*Glycation* is the result of proteins being exposed to elevated levels of blood sugar (glucose). Glycated proteins have impaired function and are broken down faster, which leads to weakened tissue strength. In the case of connective tissue, this means a loss of function, delayed wound healing, loss of elasticity, and an overall reduction in mobility and flexibility. Elevated blood sugar also leads directly to increased inflammatory load and increased free radical damage—both of which lead to further tissue damage, reduced turnover, and delayed healing.

Glycation can be controlled by eating fewer processed foods and more whole-foods (to maintain normal blood glucose), as well as by using certain glucose-control supplements such as alpha lipoic acid (also an antioxidant), banaba leaf, gymnema, fenugreek and others.

*Cortisol* is the primary stress hormone to which overexposure leads directly and rapidly to elevated blood sugar (increasing glycation), as well as increased levels of free radicals and eicosanoids. Of the four metabolic factors that influence connective tissue health, cortisol control can be thought of as first in line because it so strongly influences the direction of the other three and it serves as a signal in the body for the rapid breakdown of collagen (the chief structural protein in connective tissues).

Cortisol can be controlled by exercise, yoga, stress management, balancing protein/fat/carbohydrate intake, and by a variety of anti-stress supplements, including theanine, magnolia bark, beta-sitosterol, phosphatidylserine, omega-3 fatty acids (also an anti-inflammatory), scutellaria, ginseng, ashwagandha, rhodiola, and others.

The interrelations among these four important areas of metabolism mean that affecting one area in a positive direction generally has a positive effect on the other three areas. Even better, however, is to employ simple strategies to balance all four areas simultaneously. For example, the development (or prevention) of connective tissue problems in the joints (arthritis), or bones (osteoporosis), or muscles (fibromyalgia) is strongly linked to imbalances in all fours areas: oxidation (tissue microdamage); glycation (loss of collagen function); cortisol (accelerated collagen breakdown); and inflammation (inflammatory damage and free-radical promotion)—so the full FlexCare Program can work wonders in each area.

## Lifestyle Factors

Like the integrity of other body systems, connective tissue health is affected by our lifestyle choices. For example, one recent study investigating the impact of stress on wound healing in healthy non-smoking men found that as stress increased, so did the amount of time it took wounds to heal. Researchers determined it was the elevated cortisol levels that were most likely to blame.

Tobacco consumption is hazardous to your health in a variety of ways, including connective tissue damage (a single cigarette contains more than 100 trillion free radicals, so each puff delivers a potent dose of cell-destroying oxidation to your delicate connective tissues). A review study conducted by German researchers reported a range of detrimental effects of smoking on connective tissue health, including reduced collagen production, a heightened inflammatory response, and suppression of the immune system (which delays the healing response in all body systems).

Fortunately, there's plenty you can do to fend off these challenges. Your connective tissue regenerates itself approximately every thirty days—a bit faster in muscles and a bit slower in joint cartilage—but overall, the turnover process means that every month you've got a new opportunity to infuse your crucial connective tissues with vitality. Drinking plenty of water, wholesome nutrition, regular exercise, a few key supplements, and a healthy lifestyle are all factors that add up to total connective tissue wellness. Some evidence even suggests that massage as a complementary and alternative medicine therapy may support a healthy renewal of connective tissues throughout the body.

## Supporting Nutrients: Giving Collagen a Helping Hand

It makes very little sense for anybody to talk about nutrition or dietary supplementation without trying to put it back into the context of how it can help the entire body. For example, I can tell you that calcium is good for your bones, but without considering your intake of other nutrients (like vitamin D, magnesium, phosphorous, protein, and sodium), a recommendation to get more calcium is little more than a shot in the dark. The same goes for dietary supplements intended to support connective tissue metabolism.

The process by which amino acids are used by the body to produce healthy connective tissues is complicated. Along the way, a number of specialized enzymes and active cofactors must be present in just the right amounts and at just the right times for the whole process to operate optimally. Among these active cofactors are vitamins like C, D, E, and the B complex, as well as minerals such as copper, zinc, manganese, and silicon that are vital components of the collagen production machinery. In addition, there are a wide variety of non-nutrient factors such as bromelain, boswellia, green tea, grape seed, and gotu kola, which may be able to enhance the process of connective tissue maintenance by reducing inflammation and improving circulation. In Chapter 5, you'll learn about the most effective ingredients to support healthy connective tissue from the inside.

## Glycation Control

As a scientist, I know that micro-inflammation (inflammation on a scale too small to be seen with the naked eye) in any connective tissue can be caused by excessive exposure to both free radicals and glycation—with each leading to their own form of accelerated aging. Some of the main dietary offenders in this metabolic aging cycle are high-sugar foods (like candy, ice cream, donuts, cookies, and sugary breakfast cereals) and other high-glycemic-index foods that quickly convert to sugar or glucose in the bloodstream (like processed grains such as white bread, rolls, and instant rice). Sugar can be toxic to your connective tissues by permanently attaching to collagen fibers through the glycation process. Wherever sugar attaches, it triggers a biochemical mechanism that creates inflammation. The inflammation, in turn, produces enzymes that break down collagen thus resulting in damage to your joints, bones, muscles, tendons, ligaments, and skin. To make matters worse, glycation also leads to cross-linking of collagen fibers, changing connective tissues from soft, supple, and flexible to stiff, brittle, and painful. These stiff sugar-protein bonds form in other tissues too—like veins, arteries, tendons, and ligaments—which is why some scientists are now finding links between glycation and cardiovascular disease and arthritis.

## Over the Rainbow

In a nutshell then, high-glycemic/high-sugar/highly processed foods flood the body with sugar that then wreaks havoc on connective tissues. So that's what not to eat. But what foods can promote connective tissue health? Start by looking for the rainbow—of vividly colored foods, that is. Plant pigments don't just make foods pretty, they also make them potently nutritious. In addition to being great sources of vitamin C and minerals (necessary nutrients for connective tissue maintenance and repair), colorful foods also contain other phytonutrients (*phyto* means "plant") that possess numerous disease-preventing, anti-inflammatory, anti-aging antioxidants.

Free-radical-fighting antioxidants in colorful foods have broad benefits for connective tissues, such as reducing inflammation by neutralizing free radicals produced during the inflammatory process. They also exert other effects like strengthening the vascular system, improving circulation, and directly preventing glycation. A special type of these antioxidants called flavonoids exerts strong anti-inflammatory effects by inhibiting the cyclooxygenase (COX) enzymes outlined earlier. Remember that COX-1 enzymes are the good guys, acting to protect the stomach and intestinal lining—while COX-2 enzymes, on the other hand, are the ones that cause pain and inflammation. Nonsteroidal anti-inflammatory drugs (NSAIDs) like aspirin and ibuprofen block both groups of COX enzymes, which is why they're effective at reducing pain and inflammation yet carry the potential side effect of stomach and intestinal erosion. However, flavonoids like those found in ginger, grape seed extract, turmeric, and other herbs and spices are able to block primarily the inflammatory

COX-2 enzymes, thereby reducing inflammation without the toxic side effects common to synthetic drugs.

The richer the color of foods the better, as deep color indicates a greater concentration of these antioxidants. Select from as many different colored foods as possible—like fruits (apples, blueberries, blackberries, strawberries, raspberries, oranges, mangoes, kiwifruit, tomatoes), vegetables (spinach, peppers, squash, pumpkin, yams, onions) and brown-toned nuts, seeds, and legumes—since different colors represent different antioxidant nutrients. A good rule of thumb is to include multicolored foods with every meal and snack—at least one serving, or about a half-cup.

## Good Fats

In the last few years, considerable media attention has explored bad fats and good ones. The now-golden rule of improving heart health by reducing bad fats like saturated fats (e.g., whole-milk dairy products and fatty red meat and poultry) and trans-fats (hydrogenated and partially hydrogenated oils) applies to connective tissue health too, as long as you also include the good guys—essential fatty acids (EFAs). Research has shown that EFAs, in particular omega-3 fatty acids, provide healing benefits for various inflammatory conditions like arthritis and fibromyalgia, and that they may exert their anti-inflammatory effects by blocking COX-2 enzymes. Omega-3s are also effective controllers of cortisol overexposure and as such, can help keep connective tissues flexible, supple, and can guard against excessive tissue breakdown.

Fatty acids are the building blocks of all fats, but the ones termed *essential* are so named because, like essential amino acids and vitamins and minerals, your body cannot produce them. You must get these health-promoting fats from outside sources. The average American gets plenty of one type of EFA—omega-6 fats (linoleic acid). Yet we're often lacking omega-3 fats (linolenic acid) like eicosapentaenoic acid (EPA) and docosahexaenoic acid (DHA). Good food sources of omega-3s include fatty fish like salmon, tuna, mackerel, herring, and sardines along with ground flaxseed, flaxseed oil, canola oil, and walnuts. I generally recommend including a source of EFAs with every meal if possible, but including them several times each week is an absolute necessity. Chapter 7 has variety of excellent recipes that will help you incorporate a rich supply of anti-inflammatory fats and antioxidant nutrients into your diet.

## Don't Forget the $H_2O$

The amount of water you need to properly hydrate connective tissues and move nutrients in and toxins out varies with several factors, including environmental conditions and your activity level (which both affect how much fluid you lose as sweat). I generally suggest an intake reminiscent of the old standby: eight to ten glasses a day (which is actually based on a rough metabolic calculation of the amount of water needed to fully metabolize about 1,500–2,000 calories of energy from food). Any good, clean source of water works perfectly fine, and the National Academy of Sciences suggests that hard water—the kind high in minerals—may be even better for health due to the higher level of nutrients like calcium and magnesium that support connective tissue turnover.

## Exercise Your Connective Tissues!

You probably think of weight loss, toned muscles, strong bones, and a healthy heart when the subject is exercise, but you may not think about how exercise benefits your other connective tissues (besides muscles and blood vessels). Regular exercise can influence connective tissue health in many ways. For example, it's well known that exercise enhances circulation, and along with better circulation goes better nutrient delivery to connective tissues as well as more efficient toxin removal. Additionally, plenty of evidence suggests that exercise reduces stress, which, in turn, calms the adrenal glands and reduces their output of cortisol. This is yet another reason that exercise that is specifically directed at mind-body stress reduction (like yoga and tai chi) may have a particularly beneficial effect on connective tissue problems such as arthritis and fibromyalgia. Another consideration is that these same stress-reducing types of exercise support total-body relaxation, which can have a pain-relieving and flexibility-inducing effect all their own.

As exercise turns back the clock for muscles and bones, it may also have anti-aging effects for your other connective tissues as well. With advancing years, not only do we have fewer fibroblasts (collagen-producing cells), but the ones we do have aren't quite as ambitious as they once were. As a result, connective tissues throughout the body lose their snap and tend to break down faster. But jazzing up your daily routine with exercise and the resulting enhanced circulation brings more oxygen and other nutrients, thereby creating an ideal environment for ramped up collagen production. Increased circulation will help deliver vital nutrients through the blood to the site of collagen production in each of your connective tissues. The easy-to-follow exercises in the FlexCare Program show you how to use physical activity to increase systemic circulation and how to insure that there are enough of the right nutrients in your blood for delivery and utilization within the connective tissue layers.

One more thing, remember the connection between sugar, glycation, and connective tissue aging discussed earlier? Since exercise stabilizes blood sugar, it can also reduce the potential for glycation's inflammatory aging effects.

## Summary

There are vast amounts of scientific and medical information concerning the details underlying each of these metabolic areas—far too much to even summarize here. For interested readers, I invite you to more fully explore these metabolic intricacies and the controlling/modulating role played by specific nutrients at the SupplementWatch website (www.supplementwatch.com). The editors, writers, and scientific advisors involved with SupplementWatch make sure that the site and its recommendations are updated routinely—much faster than what can be accomplished with printed media. By visiting the site you can gain a greater understanding of the role that specific nutrients play in connective tissue health and how you can harness them for your own natural fountain of youth.

# 4

---

**EATING FOR FLEXIBILITY:
SUPPORTING INJURY REPAIR
WITH NUTRITION**

Whether you're a competitive athlete or a weekend warrior, you probably know the frustration that comes with recovering from a connective tissue injury. Virtually all forms of exercise deliver some amount of pulling, pushing, twisting, and bending to the bones, cartilage, tendons, ligaments, and skin that make up your connective tissue matrix. When traumatic or overuse injuries occur, the body mounts a repair process that hinges on adequate synthesis of collagen proteins. This chapter highlights the importance of proper nutrition and dietary supplementation as a way to support the natural healing process and help get you back into the game quicker and stronger. For many people dealing with constant pain, inflammation, and discomfort, getting back in the game might be as simple as reducing knee pain enough to climb stairs effortlessly or controlling low-back pain enough to enable you to move around freely.

Remember that connective tissue is constantly in a steady state of turnover, meaning that the collagen matrix is continually being broken down and rebuilt in response to the demands placed on it. Under normal circumstances, collagen turnover is balanced between synthetic (production) and degenerative (breakdown) processes. This allows periodic removal and repair of damaged tissue and its replacement with healthy new tissue. Under certain conditions, however, the balance between collagen breakdown and repair can become unbalanced, resulting in excess connective tissue deterioration. Sometimes this is due to extreme tissue destruction, sometimes to inadequate repair, and sometimes to a combination of both.

A number of factors are known to influence the body's ability to adapt to conditions that unbalance the collagen turnover process:

- *Aging* causes a number of biochemical and biomechanical changes in connective tissues. For example, in joint cartilage, both the number of cells (chrondoblasts) and their individual activity may decline with age. This means that cartilage in older joints may be less able to repair damage and is less resistant to injury than cartilage in younger joints.
- *Obesity* is a known risk factor for joint pain and stiffness due to the increased chronic load delivered to joints. The primary weight-bearing joints of the body, the knees and hips, are particularly susceptible to damage from excessive weight bearing.
- *Genetic factors* are thought to play a role in collagen metabolism and may explain some of the variation in risk of connective tissue diseases such as arthritis and osteoporosis.
- *Physical activity* has the potential to significantly influence collagen metabolism by enhancing transport of nutrients from the blood into the connective tissues where they can be used. Too little activity or too much mechanical stress may unbalance the collagen repair process and impair connective tissue function.
- *Medications,* including over-the-counter pain relievers like

aspirin, ibuprofen (Advil), and naproxen (Aleve) can interfere with the normal collagen repair process. Although such medications are widely used for the temporary relief of pain and inflammation of arthritis and other injuries, their overall effect is to address the symptom of pain, not the underlying cause of tissue damage. Chronic use of such pain relievers may actually accelerate connective tissue damage and worsen the very condition from which you are trying to get relief.

## Diet and Connective Tissue Repair

You've certainly heard the saying, "You are what you eat"—but did you ever stop to think that what you eat might also influence how you look and how you feel and whether or not your joints creak and ache? Based on several recent scientific studies and many decades of population studies, we now know quite clearly that nutritional factors can influence connective tissue health in a variety of ways. For example, your choice of diet can promote or prevent many of the metabolic factors associated with arthritis, osteoporosis, fibromyalgia, low-back pain, and the very process of aging itself.

## What to Avoid

When it comes to diet and connective tissue health, we know a great deal about what not to do. This comes down to avoiding or limiting your intake of highly refined carbohydrates, sodas, and processed foods containing high-fructose corn syrup and trans-fat (the label will say hydrogenated or partially hydrogenated oil). Why do you need to avoid these types of highly processed foods? Because they set off a metabolic chain-reaction in the body that leads to unhealthy elevations in blood sugar, insulin, cortisol, cytokines, and free radicals—yikes!—all that from eating a Twinkie.

Not only are these metabolic events bad for your long-term health—they're also bad for both your long- and short-term ability to heal and rebuild connective tissues. For example, chowing down on that monster-size bagel (refined carbs) leads to microscopic tissue destruction via a number of related events, such as:

- Spiking blood sugar and insulin levels lead to protein glycation and destruction of collagen and elastin (key structural proteins in healthy connective tissues).
- Elevated cortisol levels lead to imbalances in the inflammatory process in favor of pro-inflammatory eicosanoids (which leads to further tissue damage).
- Inflammatory eicosanoid signaling elevates free radical destruction of tissue membranes throughout the body—especially in the connective tissues.

## What to Eat

It's a scary proposition that poor dietary choices can lead to so much destructive metabolism in your body, but all of us make these choices many times a day (every time we eat). Luckily, we also have very good scientific evidence to help us choose a diet that provides ingredients to not only reduce these detrimental metabolic chain reactions, but to actually prevent and reverse the effects of oxidation, glycation, inflammation, and all the rest on connective tissue health.

Some of the easiest routes to controlling these metabolic marauders are to:

- Eat more of the right kinds of fats (and less of the bad kind)
- Eat fewer refined carbohydrates (and more whole grain carbs)
- Eat more antioxidants (from brightly colored fruits, veggies, and supplements)
- Reduce stress (or control your exposure to the stress hormone cortisol)

## GOOD FAT, GOOD CARBS

Based on data collected since the mid-1970s on more than 90,000 women and 50,000 men, researchers at Harvard University have shown quite convincingly that the type of fat and the type of carbohydrate that you eat are vitally important in determining your overall level of systemic inflammation and heart disease. Their recommendations focus your dietary choices toward healthy fats (olive, canola, soy, corn, sunflower, and peanut oils) and healthy carbohydrates (whole grain foods such as whole wheat bread, oatmeal, and brown rice)—and are associated with a 30–40 percent reduction in risk for inflammatory heart disease. In support of the Harvard recommendations is a recent study from Dutch researchers in the *American Journal of Clinical Nutrition,* which shows that eating more monounsaturated oils is associated with better hydration of connective tissues (which tend to have a high water content, when healthy). Researchers from the University of Colorado have also noted in the *Archives of Dermatology* the astonishing differences in rates of connective tissue (skin) inflammation between populations with a high intake of refined carbohydrates (lots of inflammation and high rates of inflammatory conditions) compared to populations eating fewer refined carbs (very low rates of both).

Modern diets supply roughly 20–25 times more omega-6 fatty acids than omega-3 fatty acids—a situation that predisposes us toward pro-inflammatory cytokines and systemic inflammation in our bodies. The best way to address these imbalances is to limit your intake of omega-6 fats (especially fried foods), while also increasing your consumption of fatty fish such as salmon, tuna, mackerel, and bluefish (which are high in omega-3 fats). For people who can't or don't want to eat more fatty fish, a daily fish oil supplement can provide omega-3s to help quell inflammatory cytokines. A number of studies have shown that dietary omega-3 fatty acids, as a direct result of their anti-inflammatory properties, can help to modulate connective tissue inflammation.

## BRIGHTER IS BETTER

Be sure to include representatives of the entire antioxidant network (vitamins C and E, thiols, carotenoids, and flavonoids). Korean researchers have reported in the *Annals of the New York Academy of Sciences* that free radicals are intimately involved in the inflammatory process that leads to accelerated connective tissue aging. Choose brightly colored fruits and vegetables, such as berries, tomatoes, and carrots, for the highest content of carotenoids and flavonoids. When supplementing, avoid megadoses of single antioxidant compounds and focus instead on selecting products that provide a balanced blend from among each category of the antioxidant network.

## Stress Less

Cortisol, one of the body's primary stress hormones, is elevated in response to stressful events, lack of sleep, and even by dieting. Researchers from London have reported in the *Journal of the American Heart Association* that even short periods of stress can increase levels of cortisol and cytokines. Elevated cortisol/cytokine levels have been associated with the development of the inflammatory metabolic syndrome that includes obesity, diabetes, hypertension, and elevated cholesterol. Effective cortisol control can be achieved by balancing carbohydrate intake with proteins and fats as well as a variety of dietary supplements such as scutellaria, theanine, beta-sitosterol, and adaptogens like cordyceps, ginseng, rhodiola, and others.

As you can see, just as we are what we eat—we also tend to feel like what we eat—and who wants to feel like junk? The solution, as outlined above, is to face the nutritional facts and eat your way to healthy connective tissue by focusing on healthy carbs and fats, controlling stress and cortisol, and getting enough antioxidants and omega-3 fatty acids in your daily diets. In doing so, anybody can truly achieve dramatic improvements in reduced pain, improved flexibility, and enhanced mobility.

As discussed above, there is nothing wrong with following a flexibility program based on just inflammatory control or on just free radical control—you'll undoubtedly see benefits from the age-old salad-and-salmon diets advocated by many nutrition gurus. However, as with all complicated scenarios in life, if your solution to a complex problem is too simple, then you're bound to spin your wheels and the results are likely to be limited. Such is the case with existing (limited) programs—while you're controlling inflammation, you're losing ground to oxidation, and while you're controlling oxidation, you're losing ground to glycation, and so on. The FlexCare Program treats connective tissue health from the perspective of metabolic control, and by doing so (addressing the cellular and hormonal aspects of collagen metabolism and connective tissue turnover) it gets right to the root of the problem.

## The Helping Hand Diet

The eating strategy that I have been using for years in a variety of lifestyle programs is not about following a strict meal-planning regimen, nor is it about restricting any foods or categories of foods. In fact, it's not much of a diet at all. Most of the people who have tried it can confirm that they often eat more food while following my advice, and they still lose weight and feel great. I call the diet the Helping Hand approach because you use the size of your hand as a portion control device. This easy-to-follow plan teaches you how to balance your intake of carbohydrates, protein, fat, and fiber in a way that considers both the quantity of food and, even more importantly, the quality of those foods.

An easy-to-follow version of the Helping Hand diet is outlined below, but for a more thorough description and answers to some frequently asked questions, refer to the SupplementWatch website (www.supplementwatch.com):

### STEP 1. CONSIDER CARBOHYDRATES

*General rule:* Foods that are more whole (in their natural, unprocessed state) are better for long-term control of oxidation, inflammation, glycation, and cortisol. Carbohydrates, in and of themselves, are not bad, but the form of carbohydrate that you choose will determine your body's metabolic response and your likelihood of being able to effectively control inflammation and repair/rebuild damaged connective tissues.

## STEP 2. PROVIDE PROTEIN

*General rule:* Any form of lean protein can be used to rebalance a refined carbohydrate. Proteins and carbs are the yin and yang of nutrition, and they have to be consumed together for proper dietary balance (which falls apart when either one is excluded or inappropriately restricted).

## STEP 3. FINISH WITH FAT

*General rule:* A small amount of added fat at each meal is a metabolic regulator. A bit of added fat in the form of a dash of olive oil, a square of cheese, or a handful of nuts helps to slow the post-meal rise in blood sugar, which in turn helps you control glycation, oxidation, and inflammation—and thus enhance connective tissue maintenance and flexibility.

## STEP 4. FILL UP WITH FIBER

*General rule:* Choosing whole forms of grains, fruits, and vegetables (as recommended in Step 1) will automatically satisfy your fiber needs. Like fat, fiber helps to slow the absorption of sugar from the digestive tract into the bloodstream. In this way, fiber can also be considered a metabolic regulator to help balance blood-sugar levels at each meal or snack. Whole-grain fiber-rich foods also contain a wide array of antioxidant and anti-inflammatory phytonutrients such as lignans to further protect connective tissues from damage.

The Helping Hand approach to eating (see diagram) considers both the quality and the quantity of each and every meal and snack, and the best part is that it requires zero counting of calories, fat-grams, or carb-grams. Why? Because the calorie-control is already built-in based on the size of your hand (Mother Nature's automatic portion control). So a person with average-sized hands will consume about 500 calories from each meal built using the Helping Hand approach. The best part is that the automatic balance between protein-carbs-fat-fiber also delivers a high degree of metabolic control, so not only are your appetite and mood more balanced, but so are your ability to maintain optimal connective tissue balance.

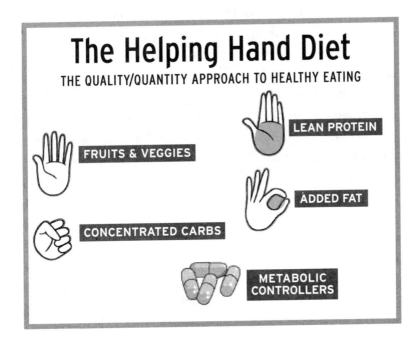

## TWO FOOD ADDITIVES TO AVOID

I'm not really a fan of the highly restrictive popular diets that cut out almost all carbs or most of the fat from your diet. These diets have poor long-term success rates and they're simply miserable to follow. As such, I don't like to tell people that there is any such thing as a forbidden food or a banned list of foods, but I make an exception for two food additives because of their extreme toxicity to the body and their dramatic metabolic disruption of cortisol and increase in oxidation, inflammation, and glycation. These ingredients are high-fructose corn syrup and hydrogenated/partially hydrogenated oils.

*High-Fructose Corn Syrup.* A sweetener made from corn, HFCS is higher in fructose than regular corn syrup or table sugar, which is technically known as sucrose. The food industry likes to use HFCS because it is both cheaper and sweeter than regular sugar, so they can use smaller amounts of it and save money compared to using pure sugar to sweeten processed foods. However, because fructose is metabolized quite differently from other sugars, over-consumption can result in some very dramatic alterations in energy metabolism, including disrupted cortisol metabolism, insulin resistance (leading to advanced glycation), and higher levels of systemic inflammation.

*Hydrogenated Oils.* Hydrogenated oils are liquid vegetable oils that have been chemically modified (by pumping extra hydrogen atoms into their chemical structure) to take on a solid or semisolid form (think Crisco or other vegetable shortenings). These hydrogenated oils, also called partially hydrogenated oils, trans-fats, or trans-fatty acids (which refers to the change in their chemical structure), are easier to handle than liquid oils during food processing, and they are preferred in many processed foods because they can add crispiness to crackers and longer shelf life to cookies. Trans-fats are known to interfere with the metabolism of cortisol (increasing cortisol levels), blood sugar (increasing blood glucose and inhibiting insulin function), and the inflammatory cascade (nudging it toward a pro-inflammatory state).

The bad news is that both trans-fats and HFCS are found in high amounts in many processed foods—but the good news is that the Helping Hand way of eating (more whole foods) will automatically reduce your intake of both trans-fats and HFCS. As a general rule of thumb, any food that lists either of these additives as one of the first three ingredients on its label should be automatically considered off limits in your quest to reduce your pain, improve your flexibility, and feel better.

## TIMING: WHEN TO EAT

The last aspect of the Helping Hand diet to discuss is timing when to eat. The approach that I have found to be most effective represents a subtle but important departure from many popular diets. Like many existing programs, the Helping Hand approach encourages you to eat several small meals and snacks throughout the day. This approach to eating can do wonders for helping to modulate your blood sugar and cortisol responses to food, thereby helping to control appetite, boost energy levels, and encourage flexibility throughout the day, not to mention reducing the damaging effects of glycation and cortisol exposure to your connective tissues.

The Helping Hand approach optimizes this approach by spacing three meals and three snacks throughout the day in the following pattern:

7 a.m.    Snack (before leaving for work)
9 a.m.    Breakfast (at work)
12 p.m.   Snack (plus exercise if you can fit it in)
2 p.m.    Lunch
5 p.m.    Snack (before leaving work or on the way home)
7 p.m.    Dinner (with a cocktail or a small dessert as your optional fourth snack of the day)

*Note:* A snack consists of one appropriately sized serving (fist-sized) from the fruit/veggie group, plus one appropriately sized serving (okay-sign-sized) of fat (such as an apple and a piece of cheese). A meal consists of one appropriately sized serving from each of the carbohydrate, protein, and fat groups, plus one or two appropriately sized servings from the fruit/veggie group.

## Summary

That's it. At this point, you can see how the Helping Hand approach to eating can be easy to follow, practical to use in your everyday life, and effective as a way to control the key aspects of metabolism related to the majority of chronic conditions facing us today. By implementing some of these dietary recommendations—and understanding how they can benefit your connective tissue metabolism—you can truly begin to take charge of your own body to reduce pain, control inflammation, and improve flexibility.

# 5

NATURAL DIETARY SUPPLEMENTS
AND SUPPORTING NUTRIENTS:
GIVING TISSUE REPAIR
A HELPING HAND

Even though a great deal of the biochemistry presented in earlier sections may appear to be a bit complicated and overwhelming, the overall picture is really quite simple. We basically want to stop two things from happening at excessive levels: inflammation and oxidation. By reigning in these destructive biochemical forces, we can slow the breakdown of our connective tissues and enhance their restoration. At the same time, we want to enhance the process of repair and rebuilding of those damaged connective tissues and also protect the new healthy tissue from future damage.

To control oxidation/inflammation, you can do so directly or indirectly (via control of glycation and cortisol). The following section provides an outline of some of the most effective dietary supplements for controlling inflammation, oxidation, glycation, and cortisol. It also provides a range of supplements for enhancing the body's ability to repair and rebuild damaged connective tissues. Luckily, the very same nutrients and dietary approaches for controlling inflammation, oxidation, glycation, and cortisol are also protective for healthy connective tissue when included in the diet after the repair/rebuilding process is complete.

# Supplements for Controlling Inflammation

## ESSENTIAL FATTY ACIDS

The term essential fatty acids refers to two fatty acids (linoleic acid and linolenic acid), which our bodies cannot synthesize and which must be consumed in the diet (vitamins and minerals are also termed essential because we cannot make them and therefore must consume them). These essential fatty acids are needed for the production of compounds known as eicosanoids, which help regulate inflammation, blood-clotting, blood pressure, heart rate, immune response, and a wide variety of other biological processes

Linoleic acid is a polyunsaturated fatty acid with eighteen carbon atoms and two double bonds. Linoleic acid is considered an omega-6 or n-6 fatty acid because the first of its double bonds occurs at the sixth carbon from the omega end. It is also referred to as C18:2n6 (meaning eighteen carbons, two double bonds, first double bond at n-6 position). It is found in vegetable and nut oils such as sunflower, safflower, corn, soy, and peanut oil. Most Americans get adequate levels of these omega-6 oils in their diets due to a high consumption of vegetable-oil based margarine, salad dressings, and mayonnaise.

Linolenic acid, or alpha-linolenic acid, is also an eighteen-carbon polyunsaturated fatty acid, but it is classified as an omega-3 or n-3 fatty acid because its first double bond (of three) is at the third carbon from the omega end. It is also known as C18:3n3 (meaning eighteen carbons, three double bonds, first double bond at the n-3 position). Good dietary sources are flaxseed oil (51 percent linolenic acid), soy oil (7 percent), walnuts (7 percent), and canola oil (9 percent), as well as margarine derived from canola oil. For example, a tablespoon of canola oil or canola oil margarine provides about 1 gram of linolenic acid.

If you think back to the type of diet humans evolved to eat (caveman diet), it provided a much more balanced mix of n-3 and n-6 fatty acids. Over the last century, modern diets have come to rely heavily on fats derived from vegetable oils (n-6), bringing the ratio of n-6 to n-3 fatty acids from the caveman's ratio of 1:1 to the modern-day range of 20–30:1— yikes! The unbalanced intake of high n-6 fatty acids and low n-3 fatty acids sets the stage for increases in various inflammatory processes, which are involved in everything from heart health to pain levels.

Fatty acids of the n-3 variety, however, have opposing biological effects to the n-6 fatty acids, meaning that a higher intake of n-3 oils can deliver anti-inflammatory, anti-thrombotic, and vasodilatory effects that can lead to benefits in terms of heart disease, hypertension, diabetes, and a wide variety of inflammatory conditions such as fibromyalgia, rheumatoid arthritis, and ulcerative colitis.

In the body, linoleic acid (n-6) is metabolized to arachidonic acid—a precursor to specific bad eicosanoids, which can promote vasoconstriction, elevated blood pressure, and painful inflammation. Linolenic acid (n-3), however, is metabolized in the body to EPA (eicosapentaenoic acid) and DHA (docosahexaenoic acid). EPA serves as the precursor to prostaglandin E3, which has anti-inflammatory properties that can counteract the inflammation caused by n-6 fatty acids.

Recent studies have shown that consumption of linolenic acid and other n-3 fatty acids offers wide-ranging anti-inflammatory benefits. This effect is thought to be mediated through the synthesis of EPA and DHA. Fish oils contain large amounts of both EPA and DHA, and the majority of studies in this area have used various concentrations of fish oil supplements to demonstrate the health benefits of these essential fatty acids. For example, one gram of menhaden oil (a common source) provides about 300 mg of these fatty acids. EPA is known to induce an anti-inflammatory effect through its inhibition of cyclooxygenase (which converts arachidonic acid to thromboxane A2).

There is also some evidence that omega-3 fatty acids from fish oil and flaxseed may help improve insulin sensitivity (thus reducing glycation) and reduce perception of stress (thus reducing cortisol exposure). A recent expert scientific advisory board at the National Institutes of Health highlighted the importance of a balanced intake of n-6 and n-3 fatty acids to reduce the adverse effects of elevated (inflammatory) arachidonic acid (a metabolic product of n-6 metabolism). The committee recommended a reduction in the intake of n-6 fatty acids (linoleic acid) and an increase in n-3 (linolenic acid, DHA, EPA) intake.

No serious adverse side effects should be expected from regular consumption of essential fatty acid supplements—whether from fish oil or other common oil supplements (see below). However, due to the tendency of n-3 fatty acids to reduce platelet aggregation (thin the blood), increased bleeding times can occur in some individuals.

The best dietary sources of omega-3 fatty acids are fish such as trout, tuna, salmon, mackerel, herring, and sardines, which all contain about 1–2 grams of n-3 oils per 3–4 ounce serving. A minimum of 4–5 grams of linoleic acid (but no more than 6–7 grams) and 2–3 grams of linolenic acid are recommended per day. Supplements of linoleic acid (n-6) are typically not needed, whereas linolenic acid (n-3) supplements (4–10 grams/day) and/or concentrated EPA/DHA supplements (400–1,000 mg/day) are recommended to balance normal inflammatory processes. Total DHA/EPA intake should approach about 1 gram per day, evenly split between the two.

The most common supplemental sources of essential fatty acids are fish oil, which is a good source of omega-3 fatty acids. Other oils, such as flaxseed, borage seed, and evening primrose are rich sources of essential fatty acids, but typically do not provide the high levels of concentrated EPA/DHA found in many fish-oil supplements. The highest-quality fish-oil supplements should provide 18–30 percent EPA and 12–20 percent DHA. The higher the EPA/DHA content, the better (but also more expensive).

## EVENING PRIMROSE OIL

Evening Primrose Oil (EPO) is most commonly used for relieving inflammatory conditions associated with women's health such as premenstrual syndrome, fibrocystic breasts, and menopausal symptoms such as hot flashes. Each of these conditions is related on a biochemical level to an excessive inflammatory response.

Sixty to eighty percent of evening primrose oil is the essential (not produced by the body) fatty acid, linoleic acid, but it is the GLA component of EPO that may be the most important for controlling inflammation. Gamma linoleic acid (GLA) is synthesized by the body from linoleic acid and comprises about 8–14 percent of the oil in EPO supplements. GLA is a precursor of prostaglandin E1 (PGE1), the deficiency of which has been documented in some women with premenstrual syndrome (PMS) and cyclical breast pain. Since decreased levels of PGE1 can increase the pain-inducing effect of the hormone prolactin on breast tissue, it is thought that it may be a primary cause of many of the symptoms associated with PMS.

PGE1 has beneficial anti-inflammatory effects, and supplementation with evening primrose oil is known to control a variety of inflammatory disorders. In a double-blind crossover study in men taking either fish oil alone or fish oil plus evening primrose oil, the combination led to a significant 12 percent decrease in inflammatory markers, whereas fish oil alone led to a 6 percent decrease in the same markers.

Evening primrose oil appears to be quite safe, but because it hinders platelet aggregation, EPO supplements may thin the blood and may increase the anticoagulant effect of drugs such as warfarin. The most common dose of evening primrose oil is 1–4 grams per day with approximately 10 percent GLA.

## BORAGE OIL

Borage seeds are a rich source of a gamma-linolenic acid (GLA) whose medicinal properties have been demonstrated in areas such as anti-inflammatory activity, immune system modulation, and management of atopic eczema (excessive proliferation of the skin cells) and other skin maladies.

Borage seed oil typically contains 20–30 percent GLA and its associated anti-inflammatory activities. Studies have shown that individuals with active rheumatoid arthritis (an inflammatory condition) experienced an improvement in their symptoms when they were given between 322 and 1,960 mg daily of GLA in the form of a borage oil supplement for six months. In another study, a subgroup of a larger sample population experienced some inflammatory relief when taking 345 mg of GLA (1,500 mg borage oil) for twenty-four weeks. Other studies in humans and animals have shown the positive effect of GLA supplementation on the stimulation of white blood cells and on the promotion of anti-inflammatory metabolites.

Borage seed oil is generally considered safe. The freshness of the oil is important. The oil contains a significant amount of polyunsaturated fatty acids (e.g., GLA, alpha-linoleic acid, etc.) that could be damaged in the presence of oxygen (oxidation) and UV light. The presence of naturally occurring vitamin E (antioxidant) in the seed can be found in the oil after the seed has been pressed. Blending additional amounts of vitamin E or other antioxidants such as vitamin C or rosemary helps to keep the oil more stable. Borage seed oil should be kept refrigerated to slow the oxidative process. Recommended doses of GLA ranges from 100–300 mg per day (one tablespoon of the oil or one to three softgels daily). There may be variations between different brands based on the extent of the oil extraction from the seed.

## FLAXSEED OIL

Flaxseed is just what it sounds like—the seed of the flax plant. The typical use of flaxseed is as a source of the essential fatty acids linolenic acid (LN) and linoleic acid (LA). Flaxseed oil is about 57 percent LN (an omega-3) and about 17 percent LA (an omega-6). LN can be converted into eicosapentaenoic acid (EPA) and decosahexaenoic acid (DHA)—fatty acids that are precursors to anti-inflammatory and anti-atherogenic prostaglandins.

Regular flaxseed consumption has been associated with improvements in the ratio of omega-3 to omega-6 fatty acids in the blood, a situation that may offer protection and relief from inflammatory conditions. A number of animal and human studies on flaxseed oil have shown a clear and consistent reduction in pro-inflammatory markers (tumor necrosis factor and interleukin).

Effective multi-gram doses of flaxseed or flaxseed oil are unlikely to pose any adverse side effects. A note of caution is warranted, however, in cases of compromised blood clotting such as hemophilia or liver disease, due to the tendency of flaxseed to reduce platelet aggregation and prolong bleeding times. A similar cautionary note is advisable for individuals undergoing surgical procedures, which may predispose the patient to excessive bleeding.

Beneficial effects have been observed at daily doses of 30–40 grams (2–4 ounces) of either concentrated flaxseed oil or whole/ground flaxseeds per day. Popular uses for the oil include salad dressings and spreads, while the seeds are often used in baked goods or sprinkled on cereal or other foods.

## BOSWELLIA SERRATA

The boswellia plant produces a sap that has been used in traditional Indian medicine as a treatment for arthritis and inflammatory conditions. The primary compounds thought to be responsible for the anti-inflammatory activity of boswellia are known as boswellic acids. These compounds are known to interfere with enzymes that contribute to inflammation and pain (COX-2, 5-LO, and 12-LO).

Boswellia sap/resin has a long history of safe and effective use as a mild anti-inflammatory to reduce pain and stiffness and promote increased mobility (without many of the associated gastrointestinal side effects commonly reported for synthetic anti-inflammatory medications). A number of studies have shown that boswellic acids may possess anti-inflammatory activity at least as potent as common over-the-counter medications such as ibuprofen and aspirin. In one study of patients with rheumatoid arthritis, pain and swelling was reduced following three months of boswellia use. In some cases, boswellia may be associated with mild gastrointestinal upset (heartburn, aftertaste, and nausea—so take it with food), but there are no reports of serious adverse side effects.

The typical recommended dose of boswellia is 400–1,200 mg per day of an extract standardized to contain approximately 30–65 percent boswellic acids. The extract should be consumed in divided doses of 100–400 mg each for approximately two to three months to achieve benefits in terms of reduced pain and improved mobility.

## BROMELAIN AND PAPAIN

Proteolytic is a catch-all term for enzymes that digest protein. Supplemental forms can incorporate any of a wide variety of enzymes including trypsin, chymotrypsin, pancreatin, bromelain, papain, and a range of fungal proteases. In the body, proteolytic digestive enzymes are produced in the pancreas, but supplemental forms of enzymes may come from fungal or bacterial sources, extraction from the pancreas of livestock animals (trypsin/chymotrypsin), or extraction from plants (such as papain from papayas and bromelain from pineapples). The primary uses of proteolytic enzymes in dietary supplements are as digestive enzymes, anti-inflammatory agents, and pain relievers.

Perhaps the strongest evidence for benefits of proteolytic enzyme supplements come from numerous European studies showing various enzyme blends to be effective in accelerating recovery from exercise and injury in sportsmen as well as tissue repair in patients following surgery. In one study of football players suffering from ankle injuries, proteolytic enzyme supplements accelerated healing and got players back on the field about 50 percent faster than athletes who received a placebo. A handful of other small trials in athletes has shown that enzymes can help reduce inflammation, speed healing of bruises and other tissue injuries (including fractures), and reduce overall recovery time when compared to athletes taking a placebo. In patients recovering from facial and various reconstructive surgery, treatment with proteolytic enzymes significantly reduced swelling, bruising, and stiffness compared to placebo groups. Similar findings have been reported for other painful/inflammatory conditions including carpal tunnel syndrome, fibromyalgia, facial bruising, ankle sprains, muscle soreness, and others.

Proteolytic enzymes are generally considered to be quite safe, although mild gastrointestinal side effects (heartburn) may result in some individuals. Those at risk for gastric or duodenal ulcers may want to avoid enzyme supplements, which may aggravate ulcerated tissues. In addition, because proteolytic enzyme supplements also tend to produce a modest anticoagulant (blood-thinning) effect, they should probably not be used in conjunction with warfarin or other blood thinning agents.

The dosage or strength of an enzyme supplement is typically expressed in activity units that refer to the enzyme's ability to digest a certain amount of protein. Because the same milligram amount of a particular enzyme may have different activity units based on its processing and blending, it may be advisable to select an enzyme supplement that employs a combination of enzymes with activity at different pH levels. Also, look for a brand that is enteric coated—meaning that the formulation is protected from digestion in the stomach for optimal delivery of the enzymes to the intestines where they can perform their actions.

## GINGER

Ginger has been used throughout history as an aid for many gastrointestinal disturbances as well as to relieve inflamed joints. The most active chemical compounds in ginger are known as the gingerols, which are also the most aromatic compounds in this root and which are thought to be the reason that ginger can inhibit substances that cause the pain and inflammation associated with osteoarthritis. For example, in osteoarthritis patients taking powdered ginger, 75 percent of the subjects reported decreased pain and swelling after treatment with ginger. There are no reported adverse effects of ginger, and it does not have any reported interactions with medications. Most studies have used 1 gram of powdered dried root per day—but concentrated extracts can greatly reduce the daily dose required.

The pungent principals in ginger, the gingerols, give it its aroma, and there are a number of other compounds present, including terpenoids and phenolic compounds, such as the shogaols. Ginger supplementation is known to reduce production of the inflammatory thromboxane compounds associated with excess inflammation and pain. In studies of patients with osteoarthritis and rheumatoid arthritis, significant pain relief is noted in more than half (55 percent) of the osteoarthritis patients and nearly three-quarters (74 percent) of the rheumatoid arthritis patients when supplemented with ginger.

## WHITE WILLOW BARK

The bark of the white willow tree is a source of salicin and other salicylates—compounds that are similar in structure to aspirin (acetylsalicylic acid). Native Americans are thought to have used ground willow bark and bark steeped for tea as a medicinal remedy for everything from pain relief to fevers. Today, white willow bark is often used as a natural alternative to aspirin and its potent anti-inflammatory benefits.

The primary active compound in white willow bark is salicin. In the body, salicin can be converted into salicylic acid, which has powerful effects as an anti-inflammatory and pain-reliever. Until synthetic aspirin could be produced in large quantities, white willow bark was the treatment of choice for reducing fevers, relieving headache and arthritis pain and controlling swelling. Although synthetic aspirin is clearly a more effective pain reliever and anti-inflammatory agent compared to the weaker natural bark extract, white willow can also serve as a source of tannins (a class of polyphenols), which may provide a synergistic action with regard to antioxidant and anti-inflammatory effects.

Stomach ulcers and other gastrointestinal complaints (nausea and diarrhea) are common side effects from prolonged high-dose consumption of either synthetic aspirin or white willow bark extracts, but lower maintenance doses of the natural bark extract are often tolerated much better than the more powerful synthetic aspirin. Individuals with concerns about blood clotting and bleeding time should use aspirin and white willow with caution, as both have the potential to interfere with platelet aggregation and prolong bleeding time (i.e., a blood-thinning effect).

For those looking for a gentler approach to balancing inflammation management, low-dose white willow may be an effective alternative to aspirin. Standardized extracts of white willow bark are available in which total salicin intake is typically 25–100 mg per day for promoting inflammatory balance.

## SCUTELLARIA

Scutellaria is also called *skullcap* and is a member of the mint family. There are more than a hundred related species of scutellaria throughout North America, Europe, and China. The most thoroughly studied, Scutellaria baicalensis, has a long history of use for treating inflammation, pain, depression, and stress. In the early days of the U.S. Pharmacopoeia, scutellaria was recognized for its relaxation effects as a mild tranquilizer

The leaves and stems (above-ground parts) of scutellaria are rich in a variety of flavonoids that have shown anti-inflammatory and antioxidant effects in test-tube, laboratory, and clinical settings. A handful of preliminary studies suggest that scutellaria flavonoids are able to reduce the activity of two important inflammatory enzymes—cyclooxygenase-2 (COX-2) and 5-lipoxygenase (5-LO).

In traditional Chinese medicine (TCM), scutellaria is used for anti-inflammation, anticancer, antiviral and antibacterial infections, and decreasing blood pressures. Three bioactive flavonoids, baicalin, baicalein, and wogonin, have been extracted from scutellaria and are thought to contribute to the major activities of the plant. All three flavonoids have been shown to alleviate the inflammation associated with inflammatory conditions such as colitis and those brought about by abnormal immune system responses.

No adverse effects have been associated with scutellaria. Through its ability to modulate both COX-2 and 5-LO enzyme activity, scutellaria is able to balance and modulate chronic inflammation in ways that drugs cannot. Typical anti-inflammatory doses of scutellaria extract are based on the plant's total flavonoid content, calling for 250–500 mg/day of an extract providing at least 60 percent total flavonoids.

## ACACIA

Acacia is also known as Cutch tree (*Acacia catechu*), the bark of which is rich in antioxidant and anti–inflammatory flavonoids and flavans. Widely distributed around the world, acacia encompasses more than 1,000 species, with Acacia catechu enjoying a long history of traditional use for treating inflammation/pain, gastrointestinal disorders, bacterial infections, and heart conditions such as high blood pressure.

Because of the rich flavonoid content of acacia bark, some researchers have investigated acacia as a potential treatment for arthritis, heart disease, and cancer (each of which have a root cause in oxidation and inflammation). Acacia catechu extracts have been screened for antibacterial, antioxidant, and anti–inflammatory (COX-1 and COX-2) activities. As an anti–inflammatory, acacia is known to inhibit both COX-1 and COX-2 activity—a potential benefit in treating arthritis without the potency (and side effects) of synthetic COX-2-inhibitors such as Celebrex and Vioxx. Researchers at the Australian Center for Complementary Medicine at the

University of Queensland have shown that acacia (used in aboriginal medicine in Australia and traditional medicine in China) is effective for the treatment of various inflammatory diseases, including asthma, arthritis, fibromyalgia, and certain infections, as well as related inflammatory diseases. The Australian researchers found that acacia was nearly as effective as both aspirin and indomethacin (a popular pain reliever in Europe and Australia) in controlling inflammation.

No side effects or adverse effects of any kind have been associated with Acacia catechu extracts—and specific evaluation of toxicity using the Ames mutagenicity test has shown acacia to be safe. Acacia may be supplemented at 20–100 mg/day and is often found in combination with a broader blend of other anti-inflammatory and antioxidant herbs, such as scutellaria, boswellia, white willow, proteolytic enzymes, and others.

## ASU's (AVOCADO/SOY UNSAPONIFIABLES)

ASUs are avocado/soy unsaponifiables—a combination of one-third avocado oil extract and two-thirds soybean oil extract. The unsaponifiables part of ASU is confusing to many people. It's a big word that basically means that this form of lipid (oil/fat) cannot be hydrolyzed any further by a strong base (hydroxide group). There are two major classes of lipids—saponifiable and non- or un-saponifiable. The saponifiable lipids can be hydrolyzed (saponified), in other words, they can be broken down by strong bases like soap. This means that the ASUs are the fraction of the avocado/soy combination that no longer produces soap upon exposure to a strong base (fat-soluble vitamins like A, D, E, and K are also unsaponifiable).

Like many fat-derived compounds, ASUs can be thought of as a healthy fat derivative. As such, and like other healthy fats, ASUs are known to stimulate collagen synthesis in chondrocytes (cartilage cells) while also reducing both cartilage breakdown and production of various inflammatory chemicals (cytokines such as IL-1, IL-6 and others).

Avocado/soybean unsaponifiables have been approved as a prescription drug in France and other European countries for several years. Lab studies on animals and humans have shown that ASUs deliver a potent anti-inflammatory effect and a stimulatory effect on proteoglycan synthesis in chondrocytes (a cartilage-building effect). Four randomized, double-blind, placebo-controlled clinical trials have been published, and the collective message of these studies is that ASUs not only have a dramatic effect on the symptoms of knee and hip osteoarthritis (less pain and greater flexibility), but also on the structural aspects of arthritis (reduced joint damage and cartilage breakdown).

In animal studies, ASUs have been shown to reduce cartilage breakdown and increase collagen synthesis in joint cartilage without interfering with the balance between different types of collagen. In human chondrocytes, ASUs reduce the production of inflammatory cytokines such as IL-6, IL-8, and prostaglandin E2. In a number of prospective, randomized, double-blind, placebo-controlled trials, ASUs clearly result in less pain and disability as well as a reduced the need for NSAID treatment in patients with arthritis.

There are no known safety issues or drug interactions associated with ASUs, though individuals who are allergic or sensitive to soy products may want to avoid them. After glucosamine, ASUs are the supplement of choice for alleviating the pain and stiffness of arthritis. Certainly, there is value if combining ASUs with glucosamine to address a range of joint rebuilding and protective issues simultaneously and from different mechanistic perspectives. ASUs have been studied at 300 mg/day and 600 mg/day doses. Both doses are safe and effective, but it appears the 300 mg dose is just as effective in relieving pain and stiffness as the 600 mg dose.

## TURMERIC

Turmeric is known by the Latin plant name *Curcuma longa* (where the name for the turmeric-derived spice, curcumin comes from) and is a member of the ginger family (Zingiberaceae). Turmeric grows in a variety of tropical climates around the world and has a very long and revered history of use as a spice and a medicinal agent by traditional healers in Asia, India, China, and Central and South America. The rhizome (sort of a cross between a root and a stem) is the important part of the turmeric plant that yields the familiar intensely yellow powder that forms the base of curry. As a traditional medicine, turmeric is used as an anti-inflammatory, antioxidant, and analgesic (pain-reliever). More modern-day research is continuing to investigate turmeric's anti-inflammatory effects, as well as its potential as a potent anticancer agent.

The primary active compounds in turmeric are the flavonoid curcumin and related curcuminoid compounds, which deliver potent antioxidant, anti-inflammatory, and chemoprotective (anticancer) effects. As such, turmeric-containing supplements would logically be expected to have a beneficial effect in treating arthritis, cancer, and heart disease.

Beyond the traditional use of turmeric and curcumin by billions of people for thousands of years, the research com-

## Table 2. Supplements for Control of Inflammation

| SUPPLEMENT | DOSE (DAILY) | MAIN EFFECT |
|---|---|---|
| Acacia | 20-100 mg | Antioxidant, Anti-inflammatory |
| ASUs | 300 mg | Analgesic, Tissue Rebuilder |
| Boswellia | 400-1,200 mg | Anti-inflammatory |
| EFAs (fish oil, borage seed oil, evening primrose oil, flaxseed oil) | Fish: 2-10g (1g EPA/DHA) Borage: 1-2g (100-400 mg GLA) EPO: 1-4g (10 percent GLA) Flaxseed: 2-4 oz oil or ground seeds | Anti-inflammatory |
| Ginger | 500-1,000 mg | Anti-inflammatory, Antioxidant |
| Proteolytic Enzymes (papain & bromelain) | 25-100 mg | Anti-inflammatory |
| Scutellaria | 250-500 mg | Anti-inflammatory, Antioxidant |
| Turmeric | 250-1,000 mg | Anti-inflammatory |
| White Willow | 25-100 mg | Anti-inflammatory, Analgesic |

munity is extremely active in teasing out the anti-inflammatory and anticancer effects of this common rhizome. In a wide range of animal studies, turmeric extracts have shown significant benefits in alleviating the pain of arthritis (naturally occurring and experimentally induced forms). In human studies, both arthritis pain and a variety of inflammatory compounds, including cyclooxygenase-2 (COX-2) and 5-lipoxygenase (5-LO), are controlled by turmeric. In a particular series of experiments at Houston's M.D. Anderson Cancer Center, turmeric extracts have been shown to control the inflammatory cascade associated with a variety of inflammatory diseases, including cancer, atherosclerosis, arthritis, and osteoporosis.

There are no known safety issues associated with turmeric. Indeed, the very long history of use of turmeric and curcumin at high levels in Indian cooking and as a spice around the world is strong evidence of turmeric's excellent safety profile. Typical dosage ranges for powdered turmeric are 250–1,000 mg/day, with concentrated extracts showing effects at lower ranges (20–50 mg/day).

## Supplements for Controlling Oxidation

Antioxidants are important for controlling the activity of the highly reactive oxygen molecules known as free radicals because unchecked free radical activity is what leads to the cellular damage known as oxidation and the cycle of glycation and inflammation that follows. When it comes to antioxidant supplementation, however, it is the overall collection and balance of several antioxidants that is important, rather than any single super antioxidant. This is what scientists call the Antioxidant Network—that network being made up of five major classes of antioxidants: vitamin E, vitamin C, carotenoids, bioflavonoids, and thiols. Your cells need representatives from each and every one of these categories in order to mount the strongest antioxidant defense.

Think of it this way. If you had the best homerun hitter in the world, yet you also had poor pitching and fielding, your baseball team would not be the best team. It's the same with your antioxidant defenses—green tea, vitamin E, pine bark, and beta-carotene are all wonderful antioxidants on their own—but combining them to create a network that works together in different parts of the body and against different types of free radicals is the most effective way to go. Some of the top picks are: beta-carotene (natural), lycopene, lutein, vitamin E (natural), vitamin C, alpha-lipoic acid, green tea, selenium, zinc, grape seed, and pine bark. There are many other choices of nutrients and herbal products and plant extracts that possess wonderful antioxidant properties, many of which are summarized in this chapter.

At the typically recommended levels, the majority of antioxidants appear to be quite safe. For example, vitamin E, one of the most powerful membrane bound antioxidants, also has one of the best safety profiles. Doses of 100–400 IU have been linked to significant antioxidant and anti-inflammatory benefits with no side effects. Vitamin C, another powerful antioxidant, can help to protect and restore the antioxidant activity of vitamin E, and is considered safe up to doses of 500–1,000 mg. Higher doses of vitamin C are not recommended because of concerns that such levels may cause an unbalancing of the oxidative systems and actually promote oxidative damage instead of preventing it. Another popular antioxidant, beta-carotene, is somewhat controversial as a dietary supplement. Although diets high in fruits and vegetables might deliver approximately 5–6 mg of carotenes daily, these would be a mixture of beta-carotene and other naturally occurring carotenoids. Concern was raised several years ago by studies in which high–dose beta-carotene supplements appeared to promote lung cancer in heavy smokers. Those studies provided unbalanced synthetic beta-carotene supplements of 20–60 mg—about five to ten times the levels that could reasonably be expected in the diet.

The four key nutritional antioxidants—vitamins C and E, beta-carotene and selenium—are widely available as dietary supplements, well studied, and relatively inexpensive. As mentioned above, there are a multitude of fruit and vegetable phytonutrient extracts available that also possess significant antioxidant activity.

## SPIRULINA

The name *spirulina* includes various species of primitive unicellular blue-green algae. These microscopic plants grow naturally in lakes rich in salt, particularly in Central and South America and in Africa. The bulk of these microscopic aquatic plants used in supplements are grown and harvested in outdoor tanks in California, Hawaii, Australia, and Asia.

Because spirulina is a whole organism, it contains many important nutrients, including all of the essential amino acids (those which the human body cannot produce), vitamins, minerals, and essential fatty acids. It also contains chlorophyll and carotenoids, both of which have been receiving quite a bit of attention for their antioxidant and anti-inflammatory properties. Because spirulina contains high levels of protein and low levels of fat, powder made from this algae is often mixed with juice as a supplement to low-calorie diets. Spirulina is also a rich source of gamma linoleic acid (GLA), an essential acid that we know possesses potent anti-inflammatory effects. Studies in animals fed large quantities of spirulina have shown that it is not toxic and that it has caused virtually no adverse health effects. Dosage recommendations for spirulina are in the range of 2–3 grams daily.

## VITAMIN C (ASCORBIC ACID)

Vitamin C, also known as ascorbic acid, is a water-soluble vitamin needed by the body for hundreds of vital metabolic reactions. Good food sources of vitamin C include all citrus fruits (oranges, grapefruit, lemons) as well as many other fruits and vegetables such as strawberries, tomatoes, broccoli, Brussels sprouts, peppers, and cantaloupe.

Perhaps the best known function of vitamin C is as one of the key nutritional antioxidants, in which it protects the body from free radical damage. As a water-soluble vitamin, ascorbic acid performs its antioxidant functions within the aqueous compartments of the blood and inside cells and can help restore the antioxidant potential of vitamin E (a fat-soluble antioxidant). Vitamin C also functions as an essential cofactor for the enzymes involved in the synthesis of collagen—the chief structural protein in connective tissues such as bones, cartilage, and skin. As such, vitamin C is often recommended for wound healing and as an added ingredient in supplements designed for connective tissue health. The combined effects of cellular strengthening, collagen synthesis, and antioxidant protection are thought to account for the multi-faceted approach by which vitamin C helps to maintain health.

In most cases, it appears that while the most important and dramatic preventive effects of vitamin C supplementation will be experienced by individuals with low vitamin C intakes, those with average daily consumption from foods may also benefit from supplemental levels. In support of an elevated vitamin C intake, an expert scientific panel recently recommended increasing the current RDA for vitamin C from 60 mg to at least 100–200 mg per day. This same panel also cautioned that taking more than 1,000 mg of vitamin C daily could have adverse effects.

As a water-soluble vitamin, ascorbic acid is extremely safe even at relatively high doses (because most of the excess is excreted in the urine). At high doses (over 1,000 mg/day), some people can experience gastrointestinal side effects such as stomach cramps, nausea, and diarrhea and may increase the risk of developing kidney stones.

Although the RDA for vitamin C has recently been raised from 60 mg to 75–90 mg (higher for men), it is well established that almost everybody can benefit from higher levels. For example, the vitamin C recommendation for cigarette smokers is 100–200 mg per day because smoking destroys vitamin C in the body. Although vitamin C is well absorbed, the percent absorbed from supplements decreases with increasing dosages and optimal absorption is achieved by taking several small doses (about 200 mg per dose) throughout the day (for a total daily intake of 200–1,000 mg). Full blood and tissue saturation is achieved with daily intakes of 200–500 mg (in two to three divided doses).

## VITAMIN E (TOCOPHEROLS AND TOCOTRIENOLS)

Vitamin E is actually a family of related compounds known as tocopherols and tocotrienols. Although alpha-tocopherol is the most common form found in dietary supplements, vitamin E also exists with slightly different chemical structures as beta-, gamma-, and delta-tocopherol as well as alpha-, beta-, gamma-, and delta-tocotrienols. Natural forms of all eight structures are important for overall health.

Vitamin E can be obtained as a supplement in natural or synthetic form. In most cases, the natural and synthetic form of vitamins and minerals are identical, but in the case of vitamin E, the natural form is clearly superior in terms of absorption and retention in the body. The natural form of alpha-tocopherol is known as d-alpha tocopherol, whereas the synthetic form is called dl-alpha tocopherol. The synthetic dl- form is the most common form found in dietary supplements, although many manufacturers are switching over to the more potent (and expensive) natural d- form.

Dietary sources of vitamin E include vegetable oils, margarine, nuts, seeds, avocados, and wheat germ. Safflower oil contains a good amount of vitamin E (about two-thirds of the RDA in 1/4 cup) but there is very little vitamin E in either corn oil or soybean oil. For those individuals watching their dietary fat consumption, vitamin E intake is likely to be low, due to a reduced intake of foods with high fat content (you'd need to eat about sixty almonds to get the RDA for vitamin E and about 400–800 almonds—wow!—to get the amount of vitamin E, 200–400 IU, associated with health benefits).

Of the different types of vitamin E, the alpha tocopherol form is typically considered the gold standard in terms of antioxidant activity, although the most recent research suggests that the other chemical forms may possess equivalent or superior antioxidant protection. Several studies published over the last two to three years have clearly shown that natural vitamin E, the d- form, is about two to three times more bioavailable than the synthetic dl- vitamin E. The natural form of the vitamin is extracted from vegetable oils, mostly from soybeans, which are cheap and plentiful in the United States. Synthetic vitamin E, in contrast, is manufactured from chemicals related to petroleum products, resulting in a chemical mixture in which only one-eighth of the mixture is the powerful d–alpha isomer.

A wide variety of epidemiological and prospective clinical studies has shown health benefits associated with higher-than-average vitamin E consumption. In most cases, the level of vitamin E intake required for antioxidant and anti-inflammatory effects is ten to thirty times higher than the current RDA levels. Although high-dose alpha-tocopherol supplements are clearly a powerful antioxidant measure, concern has recently been raised because such supplements may displace body stores of the other naturally occurring vitamin E forms.

Overall, the majority of evidence on vitamin E indicates that a balanced intake of each of the naturally occurring forms of vitamin E may be the most prudent approach in terms of overall health benefits. For example, high-dose alpha-form supplements can reduce body stores of gamma-tocopherol, whereas a more balanced intake of each maintains elevated tissue stores of both. Such findings are potentially important, given that gamma-tocopherol is the major form of vitamin E in the U.S. diet and has been found to inhibit lipid peroxidation (cell membrane damage) more effectively than alpha-tocopherol. This may mean that the different vitamin E forms may complement each other in the body.

Side effects associated with vitamin E supplements are exceedingly rare. A caution is advised, however, in those individuals at risk for prolonged bleeding, such as those taking anticoagulant medications, because vitamin E supplements can decrease blood clotting ability (reduced platelet aggregation) and prolong bleeding time.

## BETA-CAROTENE

Beta-carotene is part of a large family of compounds known as carotenoids, which includes over 600 members such as lycopene and lutein. Carotenoids are widely distributed in fruits and vegetables and are responsible, along with flavonoids, for contributing the color to many plants (a rule of thumb is the brighter, the better). In terms of nutrition, beta-carotene's primary role is as a precursor to vitamin A (the body can convert beta-carotene into vitamin A as it is needed). It is important to note that beta-carotene and vitamin A are often described in the same breath, almost as if they were the same compound (which they are not). Although beta-carotene can be converted to vitamin A in the body, there are important differences in terms of action and safety between the two compounds. Beta-carotene, like most carotenoids, is also a powerful antioxidant and is especially effective at preventing inflammatory damage. The best food sources are brightly colored fruits and veggies such as cantaloupe, apricots, carrots, red peppers, sweet potatoes, and dark leafy greens.

Evidence from population studies suggests that mixed sources of carotenoids from foods (eating lots of fruits and veggies) can help protect against many forms of oxidative and inflammatory diseases such as cancer and heart disease. As an antioxidant, it is logical (perhaps) to assume that beta-carotene (which is the primary carotenoid in the diet), may be responsible for a significant portion of the observed beneficial health effects of carotenoid-rich diets.

It is important to note that the vast majority of the scientific evidence for the health benefits of beta-carotene comes from studies that looked at food sources of beta-carotene (and other carotenoids, often referred to as mixed carotenoids)—not supplements. From population (epidemiological) studies, we know that a high consumption of fruits and vegetables is associated with a significant reduction in many inflammatory diseases. Because the data suggested that the active components in a plant-based diet may be carotenoids, and because beta-carotene is the chief carotenoid in our diets, it was widely believed (until about the mid-1990s) that the majority of the health benefits attributable to fruits and vegetables may be due to beta-carotene.

One of the largest epidemiological studies, the Physicians' Health Study (PHS) of over 22,000 male physicians found that while high levels of carotenoids obtained from the diet were associated with reduced cancer risk, beta-carotene from supplements (about 25 mg/day) had no effect on cancer risk. A possible explanation for this finding may be that while purified beta-carotene may contribute some antioxidant benefits, a blend of carotenoids (and/or other compounds in fruits and veggies) is probably even more important for preventing cancer. It may even be possible that isolated beta-carotene supplements could interfere with absorption or metabolism of other beneficial carotenoids from the diet.

Unfortunately, intervention studies that have looked at purified synthetic beta-carotene supplements (not mixed carotenoids) have not cleared up any of the confusion. In 1994, the results from a large (almost 30,000 subjects) supplementation study (ATBC—the Alpha-Tocopherol and Beta-Carotene study) showed not only that beta-carotene supplements (20 mg/day for 5–8 years) did not prevent lung cancer in high-risk subjects (long-time male smokers), but actually caused an increase in lung cancer risk by almost 20 percent. This same study also found a 10 percent increase in heart disease and a 20 percent increase in strokes among the beta-carotene users. In 1996, another large study (CARET—the Beta-Carotene and Retinol Efficacy Trial) found virtually the same thing, with subjects receiving beta-carotene showing almost 50 percent more cases of lung cancer. These results were so alarming that the National Cancer Institute decided to halt the $40 million study nearly two years early. The ATBC study examined long-time heavy smokers, while the CARET study looked at present and former smokers as well as workers exposed to asbestos—all of which can be considered high-risk populations for developing lung cancer (which may or may not have contributed to the surprising study results).

At recommended dosages, beta-carotene is thought to be quite safe—although at least two large studies have shown that high-dose beta-carotene (20–50 mg/day) can increase the risk of heart disease and cancer in smokers. Other reported side effects from high dose beta-carotene supplements (100,000 IU or 60 mg per day) include nausea, diarrhea, and a yellow/orange tinge to the skin (especially the hands and feet), which fades at lower doses of beta-carotene. The safest way to get your beta-carotene and other carotenoids is from eating a wide variety of brightly colored fruits and vegetables.

## GREEN TEA

Green tea is the second-most consumed beverage in the world (water is the first) and has been used medicinally for centuries in India and China. Green tea is prepared by picking, lightly steaming, and allowing the leaves to dry. Black tea, the most popular type of tea in the U.S., is made by allowing the leaves to ferment before drying. Due to differences in the fermentation process, a portion of the active compounds are destroyed in black tea, but remain active in green tea. The active constituents in green tea are a family of polyphenols (catechins) and flavonols that possess potent antioxidant activity. Tannins, large polyphenol molecules, form the bulk of the active compounds in green tea, with catechins comprising nearly 90 percent. Several catechins are present in significant quantities: epicatechin (EC), epigallocatechin (EGC), epicatechin gallate (ECG) and epigallocatechin gallate (EGCG). EGCG makes up about 10–50 percent of the total catechin content and appears to be the most powerful of the catechins, with antioxidant activity about 25–100 times more potent than vitamins C and E. One cup of green tea may provide 10–40 mg of polyphenols and has antioxidant activity greater than a serving of broccoli, spinach, carrots, or strawberries.

Because the active compounds, the catechins, found in green tea are known to possess potent antioxidant activity, they may provide beneficial health effects by protecting the body from the damaging effects of oxidative damage from free radicals. From laboratory findings, it is clear that green tea is an effective antioxidant, that it provides clear protection from experimentally induced DNA damage, and that it can slow or halt the initiation and progression of oxidation and inflammation. Several epidemiological studies show an association between consumption of total flavonoids in the diet and the risk for inflammatory conditions. Men with the highest consumption of flavonoids (from fruits and vegetables) have approximately half the risk of heart disease and cancer (both are oxidative and inflammatory diseases) compared with those with the lowest intake.

Green tea consumption of as much as twenty cups per day has not been associated with any significant side effects. In high doses, teas that contain caffeine may lead to restlessness, insomnia, and tachycardia. Decaffeinated versions of green tea and green tea extracts are available—but due to differences in caffeine extraction methods, the amounts of phenolic/catechin compounds can vary between extracts. Be sure to choose an extract that is decaffeinated as well as standardized for total polyphenol content and/or catechin concentrations. In addition, individuals taking aspirin or other anticoagulant medications on a daily basis should be aware of the possible inhibition of platelet aggregation (blood clotting) associated with green tea (in some cases, green tea may prolong bleeding times).

Typical dosage recommendations are for 125–500 mg/day, preferably of an extract standardized to at least 40 percent polyphenols (roughly equivalent to four to ten cups of brewed green tea).

## FLAVONOIDS/POLYPHENOLS

Polyphenols are a class of phytochemicals found in high concentrations in wine, tea, grapes and a wide variety of other plants and have been associated with heart disease and cancer prevention. Phenolic compounds are responsible for the brightly colored pigments of many fruits and vegetables, but one of their main functions is to protect plants from disease and ultraviolet light in order to prevent damage to seeds until they germinate. One of the more nutritionally important classes of polyphenols, the flavonoids, is widely distributed in plant foods and includes:

• Lignins (nuts, whole grain cereals)
• Proanthocyanins (grapes, pine bark)

- Anthocyanins/Anthocyanidins (brightly colored fruits and vegetables, berries) Isoflavones—genistein/daidzein (soybeans)
- Catechins (tea, grapes, wine)
- Tannins (tea, nuts)
- Quercetin (grapes, wine, onions)
- Naringenin/Hesperidin (citrus fruits)

Epidemiologic studies have shown a relationship between high dietary intakes of phenolics and reduced risk of cardiovascular disease and cancer. You've undoubtedly heard of the French paradox by which regular moderate consumption of red wine (which is rich in polyphenols) is associated with low rates of coronary artery disease (an oxidative and inflammatory disease). In general, polyphenols (flavonoids) are thought to deliver health benefits by several mechanisms, including: (1) direct free radical quenching, (2) protection and regeneration of other dietary antioxidants (like vitamin E), and (3) a generalized anti-inflammatory effect.

No significant side effects are evident from regular consumption of polyphenol or flavonoid-containing dietary supplements. Fruits and vegetables can vary significantly in total polyphenol content, depending on the part of the plant used, cultivation and harvesting methods, degree of ripeness, storage conditions, and processing methods. Dietary recommendations for five or more servings of fruits and vegetables daily would result in a total flavonoid intake of about 150–300 mg per day. Supplemental intake should be in this range and specific recommendations will vary depending on the compound in question (e.g., grape seed, pine bark, green tea, etc.).

## LYCOPENE

Lycopene is a carotenoid (like beta-carotene) that is responsible for giving tomatoes their red color. Although there are about 600 carotenoids, lycopene is the most abundant form found in the American diet (beta-carotene is second). More than 80 percent of the lycopene consumed in the U.S. comes from tomato sauce, pizza, and ketchup. The lycopene content of tomatoes can be influenced dramatically during the ripening process and large differences are noted between various types of tomatoes (e.g., red have more lycopene than yellow varieties). The bioavailability of lycopene is increased following cooking, so processed tomato products such as ketchup, tomato juice, and pizza sauce have more bioavailable lycopene than do fresh tomatoes.

Several epidemiologic studies have shown that consumption of foods high in lycopene (tomatoes, pizza sauce, and tomato juice) is associated with lower rates of inflammation and plasma lycopene levels are clearly reduced by about 40–50 percent in smokers whose lungs are exposed to a high degree of oxidative damage. Dietary supplements containing 20–40 mg of lycopene have been shown to reduce DNA damage in white blood cells—probably due to the reduction in oxidative damage to DNA and lipoproteins. As an antioxidant, lycopene is twice as effective as beta-carotene in protecting white blood cells from membrane damage from free radicals.

No significant adverse side effects are associated with regular consumption of supplemental levels of lycopene—but owing to the controversy surrounding high doses of supplemental beta-carotene (which appears to increase lung cancer risk), doses of lycopene should remain in the range of levels attainable from a diet high in tomato-based products (20–40 mg/day).

## GOTU KOLA

In India and Indonesia, gotu kola has a long history of use to promote wound healing in collagen–rich connective tissues such as skin, tendons, and joints. In Europe, extracts are used as drugs for the treatment of wound healing defects. Gotu kola should not be confused with the kola nut, which is completely unrelated and is often used in dietary supplements as a natural source of caffeine.

Gotu kola contains a blend of compounds including at least three triterpenes (asiatic acid, madecassic acid, and asiaticoside) that have antioxidant benefits and an ability to stimulate collagen synthesis for tissue regeneration. Perhaps the best data for gotu kola is shown by its ability to improve symptoms of varicose veins (caused by a defect in collagen turnover), particularly overall discomfort, tiredness, and swelling. In human studies, gotu kola extract (30–180 mg/day for 4 weeks) led to improvements in various measurements of vein function (foot swelling, ankle edema, and fluid leakage from the veins, all of which indicate a more robust cycle of collagen synthesis and repair) compared to placebo.

Gotu kola appears to have a generally beneficial effect on connective tissues, where it may improve the structure and function, keeping veins stronger and also possibly reducing the symptoms of other connective tissue diseases. In one animal study, asiatic acid and asiaticoside were the most active of the three triterpenes, but all three were effective in stimulating collagen synthesis and glycosaminoglycan synthesis. Radiation injury to the skin of rats can be reduced by treat-

## Table 3. Supplements for Controlling Oxidation

| SUPPLEMENT | DOSE (DAILY) | MAIN EFFECT |
| --- | --- | --- |
| Carotenoids (lycopene & beta-carotene) | Lycopene: 2-10 mg Beta-carotene 3-6 mg | Antioxidant |
| Flavonoids | 150-300 mg | Antioxidant, Collagen Support |
| Gotu Kola | 60-180 mg | Antioxidant, Collagen Support |
| Green Tea | 125-500 mg | Antioxidant |
| Spirulina | 2-3 g | Antioxidant |
| Vitamin C | 200-1,000 mg | Antioxidant, Collagen Support |
| Vitamin E | 200-400 IU | Antioxidant |

ment with madecassol (one of the triterpene compounds in gotu kola), suggesting collagen regeneration and anti-inflammatory activity.

The activity of gotu kola has been studied in normal as well as delayed-type wound healing. In one animal study, gotu kola produced a 56 percent increase in hydroxyproline, 57 percent increase in tensile strength, and increased collagen content in surgical wounds. In diabetic rats, where healing is delayed, gotu kola increased hydroxyproline content, tensile strength, collagen content, thereby facilitating wound healing. Each of these studies suggests that gotu kola may work by stimulating synthesis of collagen and increasing connective tissue strength.

Other studies have indicated an antioxidant effect of gotu kola, with results showing an increase in both enzymatic and non-enzymatic antioxidants, namely superoxide dismutase (35 percent), catalase (67 percent), glutathione peroxidase (49 percent), vitamin E (77 percent), and ascorbic acid (36 percent) in newly formed tissues. It also results in a several-fold decrease in lipid peroxide levels (69 percent) as measured in terms of thiobarbituric acid reactive substance (TBARS). This enhancement of antioxidant levels at an initial stage of healing may be an important contributory factor in the healing properties of gotu kola.

Orally, gotu kola appears to be nontoxic and it seldom causes any side effects, though there is some anecdotal evidence that gotu kola may result in elevated blood sugar levels—an effect that could be of concern to individuals with diabetes. Typical dosage recommendations for gotu kola are in the range of 60–180 mg/day, usually consumed in divided doses (20–60 mg) three times daily for at least four weeks. It is important to look for an extract standardized to contain triterpene compounds—typically 30–40 percent and including asiaticoside, asiatic acid, madecassic acid, and madecassoside (these compounds typically occur at only 1–4 percent in the whole herb).

## Supplements for Enhancing Connective Tissue Repair

There is little doubt in the minds of nutritionally oriented physicians and scientists that dietary supplements can indeed be helpful in supporting cartilage synthesis, repair, and maintenance. Glucosamine is among the most popular joint supplements. Doses of 1,500 mg per day appear to be quite safe and effective, but approximately four to eight weeks may be necessary before the joint benefits of glucosamine become evident. High levels of antioxidants in the diet, particularly vitamins C and E, have been reported to slow the rate of joint deterioration in the knees and reduce symptoms of pain and stiffness (compared to people who consume low levels of dietary antioxidants). Trace minerals such as boron, manganese, copper, selenium, silicon, sulfur, and zinc are known to influence connective tissue metabolism, and boron supplements have specifically been associated with relief from joint pain and stiffness. Boswellia serrata, curcumin (from turmeric root), ginger, scutellaria, and white willow have anti-inflammatory actions similar to conventional non-steroidal anti-inflammatory medications (NSAIDs)—but without the gastrointestinal side effects common to many NSAIDs.

## GLUCOSAMINE SULFATE

Glucosamine is an aminopolysaccharide (a combination of the amino acid glutamine and the simple sugar glucose). Glucosamine is concentrated in joint cartilage where it is incorporated into longer chains known as glycosaminoglycans and finally into very large structures known as proteoglycans. The proteoglycans function to attract water into the joint space for lubrication of the cartilage during movement.

The principle behind glucosamine supplementation is that the glucosamine is delivered to the joint space and incorporated into the proteoglycans of joint cartilage to maintain structure and repair damage. Glucosamine may also stimulate chondrocytes (cartilage cells) to begin producing healthy new cartilage matrix (both collagen and proteoglycans).

Numerous European and American studies show a clear benefit of glucosamine supplements for relief of joint pain and stiffness associated with arthritis. In general, one to three months of glucosamine supplementation seems to be more effective than a placebo and at least as effective as analgesic and non-steroidal anti-inflammatory drugs (NSAIDs), like acetaminophen and ibuprofen, in reducing the joint pain of osteoarthritis.

Most recently, a five-year $14-million study conducted by the National Institutes of Health (NIH) at sixteen academic health-care facilities and involving more than 3,000 patients, has shown that glucosamine is indeed a safe and effective therapy for alleviating the pain and stiffness of arthritis. Both the NIH-led study and a series of studies from European pharmaceutical companies has shown that glucosamine is as effective as Celebrex and acetaminophen (Tylenol) in reducing pain. The same researchers also found that glucosamine supplements are absorbed much more efficiently compared to chondroitin supplements (see below for a discussion of chondroitin), leading the European researchers to conclude that "glucosamine sulfate . . . might be the preferred symptomatic medication in knee osteoarthritis."

No significant adverse effects have been noted with glucosamine supplementation. Diabetics may want to exercise a degree of caution when using glucosamine supplements, as there have been several animal studies and one small human pilot study that have suggested an increase in blood sugar levels during regular glucosamine consumption (though most of the animal studies have used injections of glucosamine).

For people with existing chronic joint pain, glucosamine supplements are undoubtedly worth the significant benefits that they deliver. Virtually all oral supplementation studies on glucosamine have used 1,500 mg per day. While this level appears to be an effective dose, there is no information to suggest that a higher does would work better or faster—or that a lower dose would be less effective.

## CHONDROITIN SULFATE

Chondroitin falls into a category of compounds known as glycosaminoglycans—basically a long chain of specialized polysaccharides (or sugars). In the body, chondroitin is used as a building block for larger structures known as proteoglycans, which are in turn used to form connective tissues such as cartilage. Chondroitin is related in structure and function to glucosamine, but while glucosamine can be extracted from the shells of shellfish, the primary source of supplemental chondroitin is animal cartilage (typically, the trachea of cows).

For many years, critics of chondroitin sulfate (CS) use for treating arthritis argued that the large size of the CS molecule would prevent it from being absorbed into the body. We now know, however, that as much as 10–20 percent of the CS is absorbed intact—a much lower percentage absorption compared to glucosamine sulfate, as confirmed by European researchers in 2005. The theory behind the use of CS to treat osteoarthritis involves two primary concepts. The first, and most basic, is that CS simply provides the raw material (building blocks) that cartilage needs to repair itself. The second theory is that CS may block the activity of enzymes that break down cartilage—an activity that may yield benefits in reducing inflammation and protecting cartilage from further damage.

Aside from some mild gastrointestinal complaints (heartburn and nausea), chondroitin sulfate has not been associated with any serious adverse side effects. The key practical consideration for selecting a chondroitin supplement, however, is quality control—a problem that is widespread in the supplement industry. One study conducted at the University of Maryland found that at least half of the commercially available chondroitin supplements failed to supply the labeled amount of the ingredient—and some provided almost zero chondroitin.

Until recently, the scientific evidence for the effectiveness of chondroitin sulfate in alleviating joint pain has been relatively weak. In several small studies, there has been some evidence for a reduction in joint pain—but several other studies have found that over the course of approximately four months of treatment, CS was significantly superior to placebo. The typical recommendation for chondroitin supplementation is 1,200 mg per day. A large number of dietary supplements combine chondroitin with glucosamine, but it is still not known whether this combination of ingredients is any better than either supplement on its own.

## MSM

Methylsulfonylmethane (MSM) is a metabolite of dimethylsulfoxide (DMSO). DMSO is a well-known solvent that is often used topically for its analgesic (pain-killing) and anti-inflammatory properties. MSM, which is about one-third sulfur, acts as a dietary source of sulfur. Sulfur is involved in a wide variety of metabolic pathways and plays an important structural role in amino acid and protein metabolism. Sulfur is required for proper synthesis and maintenance of connective tissues such as skin, hair, nails, tendons, and cartilage. Many supplements claim MSM to be a dietary treatment for osteoarthritis based on the presence of sulfur in connective tissues such as collagen (collagen comprises nearly three quarters of the solid portion of cartilage).

Despite the wide range of anecdotal reports of MSM effectiveness, there is little compelling scientific evidence supporting such claims, particularly for osteoarthritis. The best news about MSM is that it can be considered very safe (though not very effective) when used as a dietary supplement. In rats and dogs, toxic effects are reported only for extremely high doses, which would correspond to well over 200 grams per day for an average-sized man (about 8 ounces of the stuff!).

As a dietary sulfur source (its only valid benefit) MSM would appear to be an overpriced supplement option. There are a number of other less expensive, yet equally effective dietary sources of sulfur, including eggs, meat, and fish, as well as sulfur-containing amino acids such as methionine and cystine/cysteine.

## HYALURONIC ACID

Hyaluronic acid (HA) is a glycosaminoglycan (similar in many ways to glucosamine and chondroitin) that is widely distributed throughout connective tissues (cartilage, bones, muscles, tendons, ligaments, and skin). It is one of the chief components of the extracellular matrix (such as synovial fluid in joints) and contributes significantly to connective tissue integrity. HA serves as one of the primary lubrication components for healthy joint cartilage, where it can help maintain normal joint function by increasing the viscosity of the synovial fluid and by making the cartilage between bones more elastic and smooth-moving.

Because HA is basically a long chain of glucosamine and glucuronic molecules, it is logical that it may have something to do with joint function. In the joint space (and in skin), HA attracts and holds onto water. In doing so, it keeps the collagen protein matrix fully hydrated and thus maintains synovial fluid smoothness to keep joints moving freely.

HA is found in many connective tissues, but chiefly in skin and cartilage tissue. HA is used medically to treat osteoarthritis of the knee—but such treatments are administered as a course of injections of HA fluid into the knee joint, where the HA is able to supplement the viscosity of the synovial fluid and thereby lubricate and cushion the joint. It is also thought that HA supplements, especially the newer low molecular weight forms of HA can be delivered directly to the joint space to  have a positive biochemical effect on cartilage cells.

There are no known side effects or safety issues associated with hyaluronic acid supplements. On their own, HA supplements do not appear at this time to provide enough direct benefits for skin or joint support to be considered high-value supplements. However, as a support nutrient within a more comprehensive joint or skin formulation, HA can play a valuable role in rounding out a multi-faceted approach to connective tissue support. Typical dosage ranges for HA are based on replacing an expected daily metabolic degradation of HA of about 5–50 mg. Athletes, individuals with high joint stress, and those with active joint damage may have higher rates of HA turnover and thus, may benefit from higher dosages.

## IPRIFLAVONE

Ipriflavone is an isoflavone compound that is synthesized from the soy isoflavone daidzein. The primary effect of ipriflavone is in the prevention and treatment of osteoporosis, where it has been shown in multiple clinical studies to inhibit bone resorption (breakdown), enhance bone formation, increase (or maintain) bone density, and reduce osteoporotic fractures.

The chemical name for ipriflavone is 7-isopropoxy-isoflavone and its chemical similarity to soy isoflavones (from which it is synthesized) and to estrogen suggest that it would also have an effect of building and preserving bone tissue (as both estrogen and soy isoflavones are known to do).

In the last fifteen years, there have been more than sixty human studies of ipriflavone for the prevention and reversal of bone loss. The majority of these studies have used a 600 mg/day dose of ipriflavone, showing significant effects in terms of slowing bone loss, stimulating bone building, and maintaining bone density. In a series of randomized, placebo-controlled clinical studies in Japan and Italy, ipriflavone has been shown effective in preventing postmenopausal bone loss, reducing overall rates of bone resorption (breakdown), and maintaining bone mass (while placebo groups lost significant amounts of bone over time).

Years of positive results with ipriflavone were called into question by a study by Dutch researchers that was published in the *Journal of the American Medical Association* in 2001. That study found no prevention of postmenopausal bone loss with ipriflavone supplementation, but there were some questions regarding whether the subjects took the ipriflavone for a long enough period of time or took the supplement as directed. The Dutch study also had a very high (and unexplained) 40 percent dropout rate. In addition, although the authors concluded that "ipriflavone does not prevent bone loss" the data presented in the paper (figure 2) shows that the ipriflavone

### Table 4. Supplements for Enhancing Tissue Repair

| SUPPLEMENT | DOSE (DAILY) | MAIN EFFECT |
| --- | --- | --- |
| Bone Matrix Nutrients (calcium/magnesium/vit. D/vit. K/calcium) | Magnesium: 100-400 mg; Vit. D: 200-800 IU; Vit. K: 40-120 mcb | Bone-building |
| Cartilage Matrix Nutrients (zinc/copper/boron/silicon) | Zinc: 15-30 mg; Copper: 2-4 mg; Boron: 3-6 mg; Silicon: 2-10 mg | Cartilage-building |
| Chondroitin | 1,200 mg | Cartilage-building |
| Glucosamine | 1,500 mg | Cartilage-building |
| Hyaluronic Acid | 5-50 mg | Cartilage-building |
| Ipriflavone | 600 mg | Bone-building |
| MSM | 500-2,000 mg | Secondary collagen support |

group maintained bone mass for the duration of the study. Lastly, while the Dutch researchers also claimed that ipri-flavone caused a "statistically significant" reduction in lymphocyte count (leukocytopenia), the drop from 33 percent to 27 percent is actually well within normally acceptable ranges, and in the author's own words are "subclinical" in nature (meaning that it probably amounts to nothing important).

Taken as a whole, the last fifteen years of ipriflavone research strongly supports the bone-building and bone-maintaining benefits of ipriflavone with eight good clinical studies showing benefits and one clinical study finding no benefits.

Adverse reactions associated with ipriflavone are mainly gastrointestinal in nature, with occasional reports of upset stomach and heartburn. Effective levels of ipriflavone are clear at 600 mg/day. This dose can be split into two or three divided doses. Food appears to enhance absorption of ipriflavone. Cell studies have shown that the combination of ipriflavone with vitamin K, calcium, and vitamin D may have a superior bone-building effect as compared to ipriflavone alone.

## BONE MATRIX NUTRIENTS

*Calcium* supplements are the king (queen) of the hill when it comes to bone health, but it's important to remember that bones are a whole lot more than just sticks of calcium (that's what chalk is). Although calcium supplements have been clearly shown to help reduce bone loss and increase bone density at doses of 500–1,500 mg per day, a number of additional nutrients are crucial for the optimal utilization of calcium. For example, *vitamin D* is needed for optimal absorption of calcium from the intestines as well as for proper maintenance of calcium levels within the blood and bone tissue. Elderly people are most at risk for vitamin D deficiency because production decreases as we age. Vitamin D supplements of 200–400 IU can help maintain calcium absorption.

*Vitamin K* status has been linked to overall bone health in elderly subjects, with those having low vitamin K levels also showing reduced bone density. Because vitamin K functions in coordinating the proper deposition of calcium crystals in bone tissue, it works in conjunction with vitamin D to get calcium from the gastrointestinal tract, into the blood, and then into the bones in a coordinated fashion.

Likewise, the absorption of calcium is also tied to adequate levels of **magnesium** and **zinc** in the diet. Like calcium, both minerals are found at high concentrations in bones, and are thought to help maintain optimal bone metabolism. Supplemental intakes of 15–30 mg of zinc and 200–400 mg of magnesium are often combined with calcium preparations.

Occasionally, bone supplements will also contain varying levels of **trace minerals** involved in bone metabolism. For example, **copper** is involved in the synthesis of collagen, which forms the major non-mineral structural portion of bones. Levels up to 1–3 mg per day are well tolerated and may help maintain bone health by supporting collagen production. Other minerals such as **boron, silicon,** and **manganese** play an important supporting role in both bone and cartilage metabolism, and should be supplemented in a coordinated and balanced fashion for optimal effects.

# 6

PUTTING IT ALL TOGETHER:
THE FLEXCARE PROGRAM

Whether your goal is to win the Super Bowl or just to clean the toilet bowl, you need to be flexible and mobile. This final chapter condenses down the previous chapters into a few useful pages I call the FlexCare Progressive Flexibility Program. The FlexCare Program is a step-by-step daily regimen of stretching/flexibility exercises, dietary recommendations, recipes, and stress management tips that can be realistically followed by virtually anyone.

If we were to reduce the FlexCare Program to its essence, it would look like this:

1. Perform FlexSkill movements on a daily basis
2. Engage in regular exercise
3. Eat "least processed" food and plenty of fruits and vegetables
4. Laugh more and control stress
5. Supplement with natural herbs and nutrients

## How Does the FlexCare Program Work?

Very simply, the FlexCare Program helps nourish and stimulate your body's natural process of connective tissue repair and rejuvenation. The diet, exercise, and flexibility portions of the program form the foundation that promotes a healthy balance of connective tissue turnover. Dietary supplements provide the most concentrated source of the metabolic regulators and connective tissue building blocks that the body needs to support optimal turnover, synthesis, and repair. The combined effect of exercise, stretching, proper nutrition, and supplements results in an ideal environment to promote connective tissue health.

The FlexCare Program is not only a simple and effective approach to regaining and maintaining your pain-free life, but it's also a new way to think about maintaining your body's vast array of connective tissues. The program is a step-by-step process to help you maintain an optimal state of repair of the vast connective tissue network in your body. By maintaining proper function and supporting the body's vital renewal processes, the FlexCare Program can help to delay or prevent many of the degenerative conditions commonly associated with aging, including arthritis, osteoporosis, fibromyalgia, and many of the aches and pains that we all confront with advancing years and daily wear and tear. The FlexCare Program can help virtually everyone, from professional athletes to weekend warriors to "never-exercisers." The main goal is for you to learn how you can take meaningful steps each and every day that will help you achieve and maintain a healthy active lifestyle.

The nutritional mechanism—or "how it works"—behind the FlexCare Program is very straightforward. The overall concept is that you stimulate and support the connective tissue synthesis and repair process with physical activity, adequate general nutrition, and tailored, specific dietary supplements.

## Perform FlexSkill Movements on a Daily Basis

Imagine the most complex, complicated and beautiful machine that you can think of. What would it be? A super computer or an automobile? A satellite or the Space Shuttle? Certainly these things are all very complex—and perhaps even beautiful from an engineering point of view—but their complexity, design and capabilities pale in comparison to those of the human body. The body is a dynamic, ever-changing, always-adapting collection of intricate structures and systems.

Sometimes the body works perfectly on its own—your lungs fill and empty, your heart beats, and your eyes blink—all without you having to remember to "work" them. But sometimes our bodies break. In most circumstances, the damage is only temporary because our internal repair mechanisms jump into action to fix the damage and get us back to full function. Sometimes, however, the damage persists, and there is a cumulative effect—a bit of damage here, a little wear-and-tear there—and eventually we wake up one morning with an aching knee, a stiff back or generalized stiffness through our entire body.

In order to adequately address your stiffness (and bring relief, of course), you need a comprehensive approach to the entire joint system—the cartilage, bones, muscles, tendons, ligaments and all their connections. Even though I talk a lot about the importance of "increasing flexibility," this is just one part of the overall mobility equation, which also includes improving the strength, stability and balance of the entire joint system. This is what the FlexSkill movements help you accomplish. No matter how stiff (or flexible) you are, no matter how much stiffness (or lack thereof) you have, and no

## Table 5. The FlexCare Program Overview

| ACTION | EFFECT |
| --- | --- |
| FLEXSKILL MOVEMENTS | Increase flexibility, muscle strength, and balance. Improve circulation to joints/delivery of oxygen and nutrients for connective tissue maintenance. |
| PHYSICAL ACTIVITY | Stimulates connective tissue synthesis and repair. Controls oxidation and cortisol exposure. |
| OPTIMAL NUTRITION | Supports the connective tissue turnover process. Maintains blood sugar and controls glycation. |
| STRESS MANAGEMENT | Reduces cortisol exposure and balances both inflammation and connective tissue turnover. |
| SPECIFIC DIETARY SUPPLEMENTATION | Optimizes natural metabolic processes. Helps control inflammation and oxidation. |

matter how old (or young) you happen to be, the simple program of FlexSkills presented here can help you improve mobility and maintain healthy connective tissue in the future.

It's up to you whether to perform your FlexSkill movements before or after other exercise. Sometimes, you might find that the FlexSkills will serve as a nice warmup and preparation for your walking or other activities (such as weightlifting), while on others days, the FlexSkills can serve as a relaxing cool-down (say, to jogging or aerobics). It doesn't matter when you do your FlexSkill movements, the important thing is that you *do them on a regular basis.*

As you perform each FlexSkill movement, it's important to remember that your joints are an interconnected system—a network of cartilage, bone, muscle, tendons, ligaments, synovial fluid, and blood. It is only by exercising this entire network with movement that you can hope to provide the stimulation, stretching, strength, balance, hydration, oxygenation, and ultimate rejuvenation that your joints need.

Perform each FlexSkill movement only within a comfortable range; you should not feel any pain. If any movement is uncomfortable to the point of pain, don't do it. Of course, you will want to challenge yourself a bit and provide a stretching stimulus to your joints and other connective tissues, but it is important to stay within your own personal comfort range with each movement. There are no prizes for pushing yourself too far, doing so may actually increase your risk of injury and tissue damage.

You will hold each FlexSkill movement for 30–60 seconds, so the whole series of ten movements will take from 5–10 minutes. This is certainly not a great investment of time, especially given the wide range of flexibility and mobility benefits that you'll enjoy in a very short period of time.

Are you ready to begin? Let's go!

# 1. CHILD'S POSE (TARGETS: SPINE, LOW BACK, SHOULDERS, HIPS, KNEES, ANKLES)

This is one of the classic yoga poses—a resting and starting pose that serves as the base from which many other poses and stretches emanate. We'll use it as the initial FlexSkill because

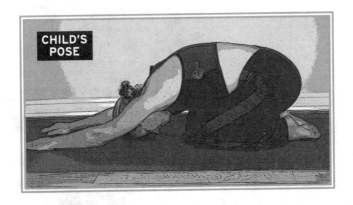

it helps awaken and stimulate each of the major joint systems that we'll target with the subsequent FlexSkill movements.

From a standing position, come to your hands and knees. Point your toes so the tops of your feet are flat on the floor and your butt rests on your heels. Place your palms flat on the mat, about shoulder width apart. Slowly reach forward, extending your arms straight out in front of you. Bend and extend your back while trying to get your forehead as close to the floor as is comfortable. When you reach your furthest comfortable point, breathe slowly and deeply and hold this position for 30-60 seconds.

## 2. ARCH (TARGETS: SPINE, NECK, LOW BACK, HIPS, ABDOMEN)

This FlexSkill is sometimes called the "Cat" and resembles a modified version of a standard yoga pose known as "Downward Facing Dog." You can move directly into the Arch position from Child's Pose, or you can pause, take a breath and start from the kneeling position below.

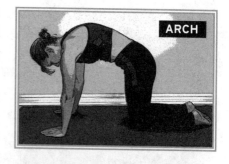

From a "hands-and-knees" kneeling position, keep your hands shoulder-width apart (directly beneath your shoulders). Slowly arch your back upward (as a scared cat might arch its back) and push your head down using a count of 5, then pausing for a count of 5 at

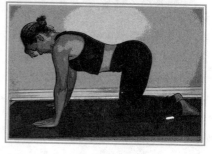

your highest arch point. Slowly arch your back down and your head up using the same 5-second count, pausing at your lowest arch point for a count of 5. Continue breathing deeply through three full repetitions of arching up and down for a total duration of 60 seconds.

## 3. COBRA (TARGETS: SPINAL DISCS, LOW BACK, FRONT TORSO, HIPS, ARMS, SHOULDERS)

This position is sometime called the "Lizard" and has similarities to the Upward Facing Dog pose in traditional yoga practice. Aside from the obvious advantage to your lower back flexibility and spinal disc alignment, the Cobra movement serves to open up and expand your entire front torso—an effect that will greatly improve your ability to breathe and thus

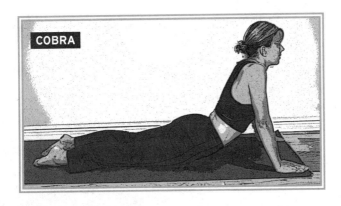

COBRA

to deliver vital oxygen to the repair process in every tissue.

Lying face-down on your mat, place the palms of your hands under your shoulders. Inhale slowly and deeply, hold for a moment and then while slowly exhaling, push up from your hands. Raise your head and shoulders and allow your lower back to naturally arch. Arch up as high as comfort allows, continue breathing slowly and deeply, and hold for 30–60 seconds. Slowly return to your beginning face-down lying position. As you become better at the Cobra FlexSkill, you will find it easier to push yourself into a fuller arch. For a more advanced movement, try arching your neck back to look toward the ceiling.

## 4. SQUAT (TARGETS: LOW BACK, PELVIS, HIPS, KNEES, ANKLES)

Okay, it's time to teach your skeleton what proper alignment looks like. This squat position is actually the "resting" position that is most natural in terms of skeletal alignment. Sitting in a chair (as most of us do for hours on end every day) is one of the worst biomechanical positions because of the extreme pressure, torque and twisting that the sitting position delivers to the back—especially the low back. This is important because low back pain affects about 80 percent of American adults at some point in their lives. The Squat helps combat back pain by realigning our entire joint system into a more natural position.

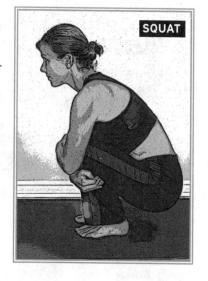

Start in a standing position with your feet about shoulder width apart and your toes pointing straight ahead. Take a deep breath and slowly squat down, bringing your butt to your ankles. Hang your hands by your sides, wrap them around your knees or use them on the ground in front or to the side for balance. Continue to breathe slowly and deeply and hold the Squat position for 30–60 seconds. As your balance improves in the Squat position, you will find that you can maintain this comfortable position for many minutes without using your hands for balance or support.

## 5. SKY REACH (TARGETS: SPINE AND SHOULDERS)

Also known as the "Pillar Stretch" and the "Mountain Pose" in yoga, this FlexSkill movement can be done seated or standing. I prefer to do the Sky Reach seated with legs crossed because I feel that I get a better low-back stretch, and because the next FlexSkill movement is also a seated position. The choice is yours, however, and you may wish to experiment with both seated and standing positions to see which your prefer.

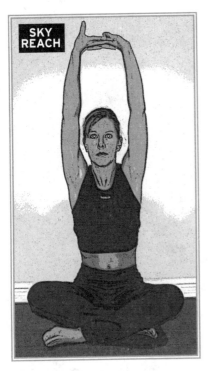

From a cross-legged, seated position (or standing with feet shoulder-width apart, toes pointing straight ahead), inhale slowly and deeply. Interlace your fingers, turn your palms away from your body and reach for the sky. Look straight ahead, spine straight, and breathe slowly and deeply. Hold your most comfortably extended position for 30–60 seconds.

## 6. FIGURE-8 (TARGETS: LOW BACK, HIPS)

Also called the "Pretzel" and the "Seated Hip Twist" in some forms of yoga, the Figure-8 FlexSkill is one of my personal favorites. As a runner and cyclist, my hips and low back are in a constant state of stress, so this movement is vital to maintaining optimal flexibility and mobility in these important core areas.

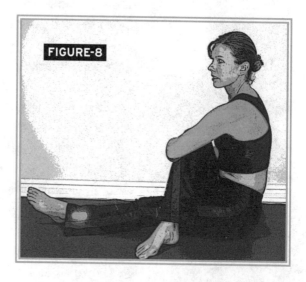

FIGURE-8

From a seated position with your legs straight out in front of you, keep your right leg straight and cross your left foot over to the outside of your right knee. Grasp the outside of your left knee and gently pull toward the ribs on your right side. Slowly pull and continue breathing slowly and deeply until you feel a stretch in your left hip, butt, and low back. Hold for 20–30 seconds. Slowly release the stretch, extend your left leg and repeat the movement on your right leg.

## 7. CROSS TWIST (TARGETS: LOW BACK, HIPS, SPINE, ABDOMINAL MUSCLES)

This FlexSkill is a two-part movement that begins with a very simple "knee-to-chest" movement you may have performed as a child in gym class. It is followed by the twisting position that is sometime called a "T-Roll" or a "Crucifix

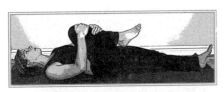

Twist" because of the position of your upper body and arms during the movement.

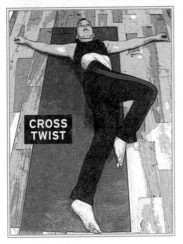

Lying on your back with both legs out straight, use both hands to bring your right knee up to your chest. Take a deep breath and with your hands on your knee/shin, slowly pull your right knee into your chest until you feel a gentle stretch in your low back and right hip. Pull as far as you feel comfortable and hold for 15–30 seconds while you continue to breathe slowly and deeply.

At the end of your hold, slowly extend your hands out to your sides—forming a "T" shape with your body. Slowly rotate your pelvis and torso to lower your right knee toward your left side—bringing the inside of your right knee as close to your mat as possible while keeping your palms and shoulders flat on the mat. At your most comfortable twist position, continue to breathe slowly and deeply and hold for 15–30 seconds. Repeat both positions (knee-to-chest and twist) with your left leg.

As you become more flexible and can pull your leg/knee further into your chest while rotating your knee closer to touching your mat, you may also begin to feel a gentle stretch in your opposite hip flexor (the front part of your hip). This area becomes very tight in many people and causes extreme strain to lower back muscles.

## 8. SUPERMAN (TARGETS: LOW BACK, SPINE, HIPS, SHOULDERS, AND NECK)

Also known as the "Locust" position in some forms of yoga, the Superman position is popular as much for its strengthening and balancing qualities as for its flexibility benefits. As a FlexSkill, the Superman movement can be performed in several variations (from easy to advanced) depending on your degree of flexibility.

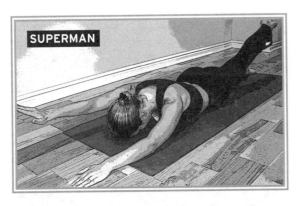

Start lying face-down, with your forehead flat on the mat. Arms should be stretched out in front of you with your palms flat on the floor. Breathe slowly and deeply for a few moments. Keeping your forehead flat on the mat, slowly raise both your right hand/arm and left foot/leg off of the mat as far as comfort allows. You should feel a slight stretch in your front torso and through your entire back, hip, and butt region. If you feel any low back pain at all, you should lower your hand and/or foot until you feel comfortable again. Continue taking slow/deep breaths and hold this extended position for 15–30 seconds. Slowly lower your right hand and left foot, take a deep breath in the beginning (face-down) position, and repeat the movement with your left hand and right foot.

## 9. PLANK (TARGETS: SPINE, UPPER/LOWER BACK MUSCLES, HIPS, ABDOMINAL MUSCLES, ANKLES, SHOULDERS, ARMS)

This movement is a classic yoga position that helps integrate upper and lower body alignment. You can think of the Plank as a static push-up in both high and low positions. We start this FlexSkill with the "high" position and progress to the "low" position. In doing so, we encourage muscle activity in all parts of the body and stimulate circulation and deliv-

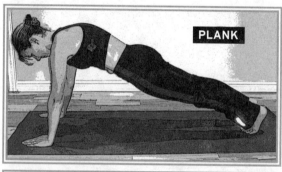

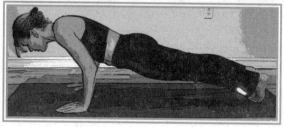

ery of nutrients to a range of connective tissues. Breathing is an important consideration in this FlexSkill—because with so many muscles being activated, you'll have to concentrate on full, deep breaths for the entire movement.

Start from the same relaxed, face-down position as the Superman movement (see #8). Place hands palm-down directly under your shoulders. Take a deep cleansing breath and fully extend your arms, pushing up to the "high" Plank position. Try to stay up on your toes while you maintain a straight spine and neck and focus your eyes on the floor directly in front of your fingertips. Concentrate on maintaining slow, deep, even breaths and hold this position for 15–30 seconds. This can be a very challenging movement, especially if you lack upper body strength, so only maintain this "high" position for as long as you feel comfortable.

You will then move directly into the "low" Plank position by simply allowing your arms to slowly bend and bringing your elbows to the side of your body. Continuing to breathe slowly and deeply, hold this position for 15–30 seconds before slowly returning to the face-down starting position with your stomach flat on your mat. Take another deep cleansing breath.

## 10. MULTI-SPLIT (TARGETS: SPINE, UPPER/LOWER BACK, HIPS, ABDOMINAL MUSCLES, LEGS, ANKLES, SHOULDERS, ARMS)

This FlexSkill is another two-part movement that targets multiple joints simultaneously while at the same time improving muscle strength and balance. The primary idea behind this movement is to get the upper and lower body connective tissues aligned and working in concert with one another. In some forms of yoga, the Multi-Split movement is known as the "Stork," the "Tree" or sometimes the "Crescent Lunge," depending on the direction of the movement.

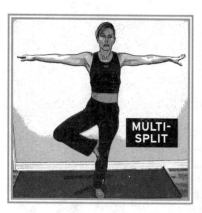
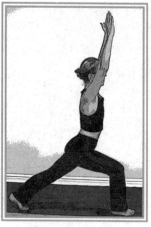

Start from a standing position, with your toes pointing straight ahead and your arms at your sides. Take a deep cleansing breath. In the first part of the movement, extend your arms up and away from your sides so they are parallel to the floor. Then, bring the sole of your right foot slowly up the inside of your left leg—raising your right foot as high as feels comfortable for you. Continue maintaining a slow, deep rhythmic breathing pattern (and your balance!) as you hold this position for 15–30 seconds. Slowly return your right foot to your mat and repeat on the other side.

In the second part of this FlexSkill, you will start from the same standing/toes forward/arms at side position. Take a deep cleansing breath, look straight ahead, and step forward with your right foot. Keeping both knees pointing straight ahead, bend your right knee into as deep a lunge as you feel comfortable. Continue your slow, deep breathing while you reach your arms up straight over your head. Imagine lengthening your spine from your lower back all the way up to the ceiling with each breath. Hold this position for 15–30 seconds before slowly returning your arms to your sides and stepping back from your lunge into your starting position. Repeat with your left leg.

After finishing this last FlexSkill movement, you should come back to a resting position for a few last cleansing breaths. You can use a comfortable standing position, the Squat position, or even the Child's Pose to bring it all together to a relaxing conclusion. Experiment with each one to determine how you like to end each FlexSkill session—or try ending with a different position each time.

## Engage in Regular Exercise

Exercise is a vital part of achieving and maintaining healthy connective tissue. Whether we talk about joints, bones, muscles tendons, or any other collagen-containing connective tissue, the right amount of the right type of exercise can help stimulate production of new collagen, removal of damaged tissue, and delivery of vital oxygen and nutrients. Just as proper exercise can promote connective tissue health, inadequate or excessive levels can likewise lead to unhealthy connective tissue by accelerating damage and delaying repair.

Our bodies are designed to move. One famous philosopher commented that the human body is the only machine that breaks down from underuse rather than from overuse (but your body can break down from overuse as well, as evidenced by the numerous over-trained athletes that I have worked with over the years). In many ways the motion of exercise or any type of physical activity can be thought of as lotion for your joints. The simple act of moving your body helps to hydrate joints and stimulate tissue repair, while the act of sitting there like a couch potato sends a constant breakdown signal (that we call atrophy) to your joint cartilage, bones, muscles, tendons, and ligaments.

But, you might ask, what is the best exercise to do? The answer is, anything that you like, whether it's the simple act of walking or something more complex such as aerobics classes or weight lifting or sky diving (just kidding). Take walking for example, a number of studies show that simply walking at a moderate (pain-free) pace for 20 minutes daily can reduce your risk of arthritis and heart disease by one-third. In one study published in the *Annals of Internal Medicine,* people who took part in a regular walking program had 27 percent less arthritis pain and took fewer pain medications compared to people who did no walking.

Walking is a pretty simple exercise, it doesn't require any fancy or expensive equipment, and you can do it virtually anywhere. That said, you'll want to make sure that you have a pair of comfortable and supportive shoes as well as a thumbs-up from your personal health-care provider that it's okay for you to engage in a moderate to vigorous exercise regimen.

In good weather, you can walk outside and enjoy the sights and sounds of your own neighborhood or a local park. In bad weather, you can walk around the mall (many shopping malls have organized walking groups that meet before the stores open and the mall gets crowded with shoppers). When you get comfortable with walking on a regular basis, you can vary the route and intensity (walking faster or slower and adding hills or flats). Walking can also be as much a part of your mental exercise as it is for your physical exercise because it can allow you time to get away and de-stress while your mind (and body) wanders.

## Eat the Least Processed Foods and Plenty of Fruits and Vegetables

A significant portion of the FlexCare Program is devoted to proper dietary support of the connective tissue repair process. Why focus on nutrition to control pain and stiffness? Because research is telling us that the kitchen cupboard may hold more effective (and safer) treatments than the medicine cabinet. This research shows us quite clearly that there is a direct link between the foods we eat and the amount of inflammation and pain that those foods generate in our bodies. The good news is that combining the right foods and cutting back on others can provide much of the pain and inflammation control—but with none of the adverse side effects—associated with drugs. The focus in hundreds of research laboratories and medical clinics around the world is now on identifying foods and supplements that can control painful inflammation and get you back to full function.

When it comes to harnessing your diet for pain and inflammation control, there are five simple steps:

## 1. HELPING HAND DIET

As outlined in Chapter 4, the Helping Hand diet is an approach to building your daily nutritional plan without counting calories, or carbs, or grams of fat, or anything else. If you use the Helping Hand way to guide your food choices, then you will automatically be eating an appropriate combination of calories, carbohydrates, protein, fat, and fiber to help rebalance your body's natural inflammatory process. Arthritis researchers in Boston have shown that excess body weight and excess calorie intake dramatically increases the risk of arthritis and other inflammatory diseases—with a 60 percent increase in risk for those consuming more than 2,100 calories daily, which is well below the amount associated with an increase in inflammatory problems.

## 2. EAT MORE FISH (OR OMEGA-3 SUPPLEMENTS)

A great deal of research over the last decade shows us that specialized fats (called omega-3 fatty acids) found in certain fish and nuts can reduce inflammation and pain. Studies from

Harvard University, the University of Washington, and many other research centers around the world prove that eating fish just once or twice a week can cut your risk of painful arthritis and other inflammatory diseases by almost 25 percent! Eating fish more than twice a week cuts risk even more—up to about 45 percent! The best food sources of these anti-inflammatory omega-3 fats are the fattier cold-water fish such as salmon, mackerel, tuna, and sardines, but you can also find rich sources of omega-3s in nuts such as walnuts and flaxseeds as well as in dark green veggies like spinach.

## 3. IDENTIFY PROBLEM FOODS

Just as some foods are known to reduce inflammation and relieve pain, some people may discover that certain foods can increase their inflammatory symptoms by causing more pain and stiffness a few hours after eating them. For example, although some arthritis sufferers find that they are sensitive to foods in the nightshade family such as tomatoes, eggplant, bell peppers, and potatoes (because they contain solanine, which may be hard for some people to break down), other people seem to be able to eat large quantities of these foods with no increase in pain or inflammation.

There is certainly a great deal of folklore and many old wive's tales about what foods might be good or bad for people with arthritis, but the only accurate way to find out your own specific food intolerances is to keep a daily food diary. Take a week or so to write down the foods you eat, the stresses you encounter, and the activities you do—and how you feel in response—and soon you can begin to notice any patterns that might alert you to problem foods. Although each one of us will have different food sensitivities, some people will notice that corn and wheat (especially when highly refined) may pose inflammatory issues, while others may find that they experience more pain and stiffness after eating other foods such as bacon, milk, beef, tomatoes, butter, sugar, or coffee. Whatever foods you identify as being linked with flare-ups of inflammation and pain should go on your own personal list of foods to watch out for. Depending on your degree of sensitivity, you may want to completely avoid your problem foods (such as switching from coffee to tea) or cut back on your intake of the offending food (such as switching from refined wheat to whole-grain wheat products).

## 4. DRINK MORE WATER

If you had to identify the most important nutrient in our diets, the carbs and protein and fat that get so much media attention would not even come close to the importance of plain old pure water for its role in long-term health, pain control, and life itself. Water is the only nutrient that we can't do without for more than a few days—we can skip our intake of the others (and still survive) for days and even weeks. Think about how vital water is to the makeup of our bodies. Our blood is 90 percent water; muscles and skin are about 70 percent water; joint cartilage is more than 30 percent water (when healthy); and even our bones contain about 10 percent water.

Your mother probably told you to drink eight glasses (64 ounces) of water daily. This is just the amount that you need for proper hydration of tissues and adequate kidney filtration of wastes out of your blood. If you exercise at all, then you need more. If you live in a dry environment (as I do in Utah), then you need even more. If you're in a state of unbalanced inflammation, stiffness, and pain, then you are very likely to be slightly to moderately dehydrated and thus have a need to drink more water to bring your state of tissue hydration back up to normal.

In your blood, water obviously serves as a solvent for vitamins, minerals, and other nutrients, helping to deliver them to the tissues where they can do some good. Water also helps to lubricate muscles, tendons, ligaments, and joint cartilage and serves as a shock absorber in bones and joints. Tissues that experience even a small degree of dehydration become less effective shock absorbers, are less able to remove toxins, are less efficient at repairing damage, and generally become more brittle and less flexible. When you're not delivering enough water to your connective tissues, they literally dry up at a cellular level and biochemical and metabolic processes simply lose efficiency.

The general rule of thumb with water consumption and daily hydration maintenance is to drink even when you're not thirsty. If you wait until you feel thirsty, then it's too late—you're already dehydrated enough to compromise your connective tissue metabolism. One of the most effective ways to maintain your connective tissue hydration is to carry a water bottle with you and sip from it at every opportunity throughout the day. You will literally be able to feel the difference in your flexibility and level of general pain between being hydrated (less pain) and being dehydrated (more pain). To give you a personal example, I do a lot of writing and speaking about the value of natural approaches to health—and a water bottle is a constant companion. When I write, I make it a point to take a sip of water at the end of every paragraph, and when I give a presentation, I make it a point to take a sip of water after every few slides. Many of my students will follow suit; it's actually a bit funny to see a room full of fifty or a hundred students reach for their water bottles at the same time as I reach for mine between slides. But what they have learned, and are putting into practice, is an important step in attaining the flexibility and health that they're looking for. You should determine similar types of water breaks that will work for your own daily activities.

## 5. SPICE THINGS UP

Studies abound demonstrating the anti-inflammatory and antioxidant effects of certain spices that have been part of our traditional diets for thousands of years. Whether we're talking about the ginger and turmeric of Indian cooking, the cayenne of South American cuisine, or the chili and other fire peppers of Asian fare, the research results are clear about the ability of these spices to reduce pain, inflammation, and stiffness when they are included in your diet. In studies from around the world, as little as six weeks of adding anti-inflammatory spices, such as ginger, to your diet results in less pain and greater mobility in about two-thirds of users. Adding these spices to your diet couldn't be simpler—you can just add them to your existing recipes based on your tolerance for spiciness. Some studies even suggest that the spicier the food, the better for immediate pain relief due to the endorphin effect. Chomping into a spicy jalapeño pepper temporarily burns your tongue, but in response, your brain releases the feel-good and anti-pain endorphins that can lessen the pain in your knee or low back for hours.

## Laugh More and Control Stress

The importance of controlling stress and exposure to cortisol (the primary stress hormone) cannot be overemphasized. As explained earlier, cortisol overexposure accelerates the breakdown process in joint cartilage (increasing the risk of arthritis), in bones (osteoporosis), muscles (fibromyalgia), and virtually every other tissue (including the destruction of brain neurons, which leads to depression). Just about the only tissue that doesn't respond to the breakdown signal is your fat, where cortisol is perceived as a potent storage signal that leads to rapid accumulation of belly fat.

Research studies are quite clear on the fact that reducing stress also reduces overall cortisol exposure, and reducing cortisol exposure is a good thing for your long-term connective tissue health. That's all well and good, but I also understand that telling you to control stress is a lot easier than actually controlling stress in your frantic life. It might help to understand that you're not alone in this regard. Do you think it's a coincidence that more Americans rate stress as the number-one reason for a trip to the doctor, while medical surveys clearly show that men show up most often at the doc with low-back pain while women tend to report fibromyalgia? That's not a coincidence, that's direct evidence that our stressed-out lives are causing us to hurt! The stress/cortisol exposure that we're awash in every day eventually shows itself as outright tissue damage—and we need to do something about it.

The FlexSkill movements, the Helping Hand diet, and the physical activity that you'll be doing as part of the FlexCare Program will all help to control stress and reduce cortisol exposure. Even letting your mind go for the 5–10 minutes that you're performing the FlexSkill movements will be beneficial for stress control. The Helping Hand diet will help take the guesswork and associated stress out of meal planning and calorie counting. The physical activity—whether it's walking or another form of exercise—should be viewed as time that you're investing in mental and physical health. You should do something on as many days of the week as you possibly can. You should also keep in mind that stress is a very individualized phenomenon, so what stresses you out might be no big deal to someone else (and vice-versa). This makes your approach to stress management a very personal and individualized process that requires you to identify your own specific stressors and your own specific solutions to those stressful events.

Whenever I give a public seminar on stress and cortisol, I like to start off by holding up a glass of water and asking the audience to guess how much it weighs. People will generally call out guesses from 6 to 20 ounces—but the point I like to make is that the actual weight of the water glass doesn't matter. As a stress to my arm, the weight of the water glass is less important than the duration of time that I need to hold it up. If I hold the glass for a minute or two, then it's not much of a stress at all, but if you asked me to hold it for an hour or a day or a week, then I'd be in trouble. It works the same way with your exposure to other stressors, such as traffic and bills and family commitments and the millions of other little stresses that we encounter day in and day out. Eventually, you will reach the breaking point—unless you actively manage those stresses. Everybody, no matter how tough you think you are, no matter how resistant to stress you think you are, no matter how much you think that you thrive on stress—

## Stress Relief: A Few Words of Wisdom

For a fun take on stress, here are a few witty quotations I have picked up from various places (and hopefully at least a few of them will make you chuckle):

1.  Accept that some days you're the pigeon, and some days you're the statue.
2.  Always keep your words soft and sweet, just in case you have to eat them.
3.  If you can't be kind, at least have the decency to be vague.
4.  Never put both feet in your mouth at the same time, because then you won't have a leg to stand on.
5.  Nobody cares if you can't dance well. Just get up and dance.
6.  Since it's the early worm that gets eaten by the bird, sleep late.
7.  The second mouse gets the cheese.
8.  You may be only one person in the world, but you may also be the world to one person.
9.  A truly happy person is one who can enjoy the scenery on a detour.
10. We could learn a lot from crayons. Some are sharp, some are pretty, and some are dull. Some have weird names, and all are different colors, but they all have to live in the same box.

everybody has their own personal breaking point when it comes to stress exposure. By using stress management, exercise, nutrition, supplementation, and periodic evaluation, you can continually manage your own individual stress load and hopefully keep that stress breaking point at bay.

Okay, back to my glass of water. Let's say that I'm asked to hold the water glass for a week. Impossible you might say. Not so, because if I'm smart about managing this stress, I might be able to handle it. Maybe I can take short breaks, where I put the glass down for a few minutes each hour.

Perhaps I can lessen my personal burden by asking a colleague or a friend or family member to hold the glass for a little while. Maybe I can leave the glass at work and not worry about dragging this burden home with me. Any and all of these (and dozens of others that you might come up with) are ways in which we can short-circuit the stress response—even if just for a few minutes.

## Supplement with Natural Herbs and Nutrients

With approximately two-thirds of the American population taking at least one form of dietary supplement on a regular basis, the chances that you're a supplement user are pretty good. You may be among the millions of people who use daily supplements as dietary insurance, or perhaps you know a little bit more about nutrition and you follow a more specific regimen. Whatever your present state of dietary practice or nutritional knowledge, the FlexCare Program can help you get started on the right nutritional path (with your food choices), but you can also fine-tune or customize your own personal supplement regimen to maximize your benefits.

Because each individual is different and may benefit to a greater or lesser degree from a particular supplement regimen, it is important to investigate the pros and cons of any natural option. In addition to the extensive outline of effective supplements found in Chapter 5, I also highly recommend visiting the SupplementWatch website (www.supplementwatch.com) as one of the best sources of information on what supplements are worth trying (or avoiding). As one of the original founders of SupplementWatch back in 1999, and

as its current editor in chief, I feel that it's importar
vide as much information to consumers as possible so
can make informed and educated decisions about which natural options might be the most appropriate for their own
unique and personal situation.

There are literally dozens of joint-support ingredients and
hundreds of combinations of these ingredients in commercial
products, so even choosing a particular product can be a
mind-boggling exercise. This book, as well as the
SupplementWatch website, can help you weigh the benefits
and drawbacks of various supplement ingredients and finished products and help you select the right product for your
particular needs and goals. For example, whether you're looking for a product that targets inflammation only, or one that
focuses on rebuilding joint cartilage or bone tissue, or perhaps
one that addresses stiffness in muscles and tendons after exercise (or even all of these effects together in a combination of
products), the information in this book and at
SupplementWatch.com can help you make the best decision
for your own personal needs.

## Summary

There you have it. I think that you'll agree that the
FlexCare Program is easy to follow and is unlikely to pose an
additional burden to your already busy life (nobody needs
another source of stress). I think that you will also agree, that
after giving the FlexCare Program a try—even for a few
days—you'll begin to feel better. In a very short period of
time, you'll start to enjoy a greater degree of flexibility, a
wider range of motion and mobility, and perhaps most

importantly, you'll be moving around with less pain and stiffness (just like the old days). Isn't that what you wanted out of the program in the first place?

I'm glad that the FlexCare Program can deliver many of the pain-controlling, stiffness-reducing, and flexibility-enhancing needs that so many Americans are struggling with on a daily basis—so I'll leave you with one simple request. If you find that the FlexCare Program works as well for you as it has for so many others to improve flexibility and mobility, then I would appreciate you sharing the program with a friend, family member, or co-worker. Think back to your own pre-FlexCare days and recall how stiff, inflexible, and immobile you were—and then think about how much relief the program brought to your daily existence. You'll be doing someone a favor by sharing the FlexCare Program with them—and they will thank you for it.

# 7

## RECIPES

Here is an entire week of delicious breakfast, lunch, and dinner recipes, with seven recipes for each meal. The goal in creating each meal has been to incorporate as many aspects of inflammation-friendly nutrients as possible. Feel free to mix and match them each day to your own tastes—and when you can't treat yourself to one of these outstanding meals, keep the Helping Hand rules in mind and combine your carbs/fats/proteins accordingly.

These recipes come to us specially crafted by New York City chef Michael Saccone. Since age fourteen, Michael Saccone has worked for many restaurants, catering companies, and clubs. Most notably, he apprenticed at George Perrier's Le Bec Fin in Philadelphia, worked at the four-star Le Cirque in New York City, and privately for several high-profile clients. As a private chef, he has gained experience in health-conscious cooking. Currently he is employed by Maury Povich at his eponymous television program and in the family home. Michael is also the owner of City Chef Corporation, which produces prepared side dishes that accompany meats, poultry, and seafood for Manhattan's top specialty markets. Michael lives in New York City with his wife, Adrienne, and two children, Catherine and Elizabeth.

*Bon appetit!*

# Breakfast Menu

## OATMEAL BLUEBERRY PANCAKES WITH ALMOND BUTTER

*Pancakes made with oats, some flour, buttermilk, dense with blueberries, and topped with butter creamed with sweetened almond paste.*

1/2 cup all-purpose flour
1 cup rolled oats
1/2 tablespoon baking powder
1/2 tablespoon baking soda
1/2 teaspoon salt
1-1/2 cups buttermilk or milk
2 tablespoons peanut oil
3 eggs, separated
1 pint blueberries
1/2 stick soft butter
2 ounces almond paste or marzipan

Grind almond paste into butter in a bowl with the back of a spoon or in a food processor until well incorporated and smooth. Set aside.

Sift together dry ingredients. In large bowl, beat yolks and gradually add peanut oil and then buttermilk. Beat egg whites to soft peaks. Start to heat grill pan or skillet over medium heat.

Gradually stir dry ingredients to yolk mixture, stopping

when ingredients are just combined. Fold in beaten whites, starting with a little to lighten the mixture and then the rest. Fold in blueberries.

Test skillet with drop of water (it should sizzle, not instantly evaporate) and add about a teaspoon of butter to pan, swirling it to coat entire surface. When the butter is sizzling but not yet brown, ladle out the pancake batter. The pancakes should look firm and have well-formed dimples when you flip them. Brown flipped side and serve hot with almond butter spread over the cakes like toast.

## SMOKED SALMON AND ARUGULA OMELET

*Omelet stuffed with smoked salmon and peppery arugula sautéed with Bermuda onion. Makes one large omelet for two.*

olive oil
1 small Bermuda onion
1 bunch Arugula
1/2 tablespoon capers
1 pinch red pepper flakes
4 large eggs
1 tablespoon milk
1/2 teaspoon salt
4 ounces smoked salmon

Skin onion, remove core, cut in half, and slice eighth-inch slices. Place sauté pan over medium heat, add about half table-spoon of olive oil and onions and start to cook them until soft flipping occasionally, about four minutes.

Trim stems from arugula, wash in large bowl with cold water, remove leaves and shake off water. Turn up the heat on the onions, add a little more olive oil if necessary, and the red pepper flakes, capers, and arugula with a pinch of salt. Cook greens until wilted, tossing frequently, until greens wilt, about a minute. Place mixture into a bowl with a strainer and wipe pan with a paper towel and return to heat, reducing flame to medium.

Scramble eggs with milk and salt. Add about another half tablespoon of olive oil to pan and swirl around. When a test drop of water sputters, add eggs to pan, let the eggs start to set a few seconds, and stir gently with a spatula, allowing eggs to set a little again before stirring again. When eggs are about two-thirds cooked, reduce heat to low and allow omelet to take shape. Place greens mixture up the center from 12 to 6 o'clock and top with salmon. When eggs are done, flip one side over and slide omelet onto serving dish.

## SWEET BREAKFAST BISCUITS AND GINGERED PRUNES

*Breakfast "cookies" made with toasted millet and eaten with stewed gingered prunes.*

### FOR BISCUITS:
1/4 cup hulled millet seeds
2/3 cup water
1 cup all-purpose flour
2 teaspoons baking powder
1/3 cup sugar
4 tablespoons butter
1 egg
1 teaspoon vanilla

Toast millet in pan over medium low heat until golden and starting to pop. Add water, cover pan, and reduce heat to low, cooking until liquid is gone, about 15 minutes.

Cream butter and sugar, add egg and vanilla. Sift together flour and powder into butter mixture. Stir in millet.

Place spoonfuls of mixture on sheet pan lightly coated with nonstick spray or parchment paper. Bake for about 12 minutes or until golden. Let cool on sheet.

### FOR PRUNES:
1 cup pitted prunes
1-1/2 pieces ginger
water

Slice ginger in half and add to small saucepan with prunes. Add enough water to just cover and bring to a gentle simmer. Cook for 20 minutes, transfer to a bowl, and refrigerate until cool and thick syrup forms, about 3 hours.

## CRUNCHY YOGURT PARFAIT

*Parfait made with alternating layers of berries, vanilla yogurt, and granola. Serves two.*

1/2 pint blueberries
1/2 pint raspberries
2 tablespoons honey
2 granola bars, crumbled
1 cup low-fat vanilla yogurt

In separate bowls, place berries with one tablespoon honey in each. Stir to coat well and place in refrigerator for 1 hour, gently stirring every 15 minutes.

In two parfait cups or tall glasses place alternating layers starting with yogurt, sprinkle with granola, blueberries, yogurt, granola, raspberries, yogurt, and a final sprinkle of granola.

## BUCKWHEAT HAZELNUT MUFFINS

*One of my personal breakfast favorites, these muffins are made with buckwheat flour and flavored with hazelnut, orange, and raisins. Makes twelve muffins.*

3/4 cup raisins
1 orange
1 cup blanched hazelnuts
1-1/4 cup all-purpose flour
1 cup buckwheat flour
1 tablespoon baking powder
1/2 tablespoon baking soda
1 teaspoon salt
1/4 teaspoon ground clove
6 tablespoons butter
1/2 cup sugar
2 eggs
1/2 cup sour cream

Set oven to 375°F. In a microwave-safe bowl, zest and juice orange, add raisins, cover with plastic, and microwave 30 seconds. Let sit to allow raisins to plump. Toast hazelnuts on a sheet pan in oven.

Sift dry ingredients together. Cream butter and sugar until fluffy and add one egg at a time, letting first egg fully incorporate before adding the second. Add sour cream and raisin mixture. Stir in dry ingredients until just uniformly mixed. Fold in hazelnuts.

Fill paper-lined muffin tin three-quarters for each muffin. Bake about 15 minutes or until golden. Let cool in pan.

## PARMESAN FLORENTINE EGGS

*Whole-grain toast slice topped with sautéed spinach, red peppers, sliced olives, and finished with gratined eggs. Serves two.*

2 bunches leaf spinach
1 sweet red pepper
1/4 cup pitted Alfonzo olives
1 small shallot
olive oil
4 eggs
1 teaspoon vinegar
3 ounces parmesan cheese, grated
2 slices seven-grain bread

Trim stems from spinach and place in large bowl filled with cold water. Lift leaves out and place in colander. Drain water, rinse bowl of sand and repeat.

Cut pepper in half. Remove stem, seeds, and ribs and slice halves into eighth-inch pieces.

Drain olives and cut into quarters. Peel shallot and mince.

Fill shallow pan with water and bring to a simmer. Add vinegar and crack eggs, gently releasing the egg into the water as close to the surface as possible. Poach the eggs until done as desired.

While eggs poach, heat sauté pan over high heat, add about a half tablespoon of olive oil, and add peppers. Sauté until soft, add shallot, and cook another 30 seconds, tossing continuously. Add spinach and toss until wilted. Season with salt and pepper. Transfer to a bowl with a strainer in it and allow to drain.

Toast bread on sheet pan under broiler, flipping to toast both sides. Place half the spinach mixture on each slice, making sure to cover bread completely. Next place two poached eggs on top of each bed of spinach mixture. Sprinkle with cheese and slide pan under the broiler again until cheese browns, about 30 seconds.

## GARDEN FRITTATA

*Frittata crowded with broccoli, tomato, chard, and red onion, and bound with a bit of whole wheat pasta. Serves four.*

8 large eggs
2 ounces dry soba noodles
1 cup broccoli florets
1 bunch Swiss chard, trimmed and washed
1 tomato
1 yellow pepper
1 red onion
1 clove garlic, minced
1/8 teaspoon red pepper flakes
salt
olive oil

Set oven to 350°F. Bring a medium pot of water to a boil. Add enough salt so it almost tastes like the ocean. Fill a large bowl with ice water. Cook broccoli in boiling, salted water until tender, about 2–3 minutes. Pull out of water with a slotted spoon or spider, and plunge directly into ice water. Repeat with Swiss chard. Drain and set aside. Cook soba in salt water and drain, set aside.

Remove stem end from tomato and cut in half east-west. With fingers, poke out seeds while giving each tomato half a light squeeze. Chop tomato in half-inch pieces. Cut pepper in half, remove stem, seeds, and ribs. Cut into eighth-inch slices. Cut onion in half, skin, remove stem end, and cut eighth-inch slices. Scramble the eggs.

Heat 9-inch sauté pan over medium heat (nonstick works

best). Add about half a tablespoon of olive oil and onions. Sauté about 3 minutes and add peppers. When peppers are soft, add garlic, cook another 30 seconds, then add tomato, broccoli, Swiss chard, and soba noodles. Season aggressively with salt and stir in beaten eggs. Turn heat to low and let cook about 2 minutes. Slide pan into oven and bake until set, about 30 minutes.

When done, slide frittata out of pan and onto serving platter. Cut into quarters and serve.

# Lunch Menu

## CURRY CHICKEN SALAD

*Tender Boston lettuce and curried chicken sweetened with green apples, raisins, and walnuts. Serves four.*

2 lbs chicken thighs
1/2 onion chopped in quarters
1 celery stalk chopped in quarters
1 carrot chopped in quarters
1 bay leaf
4 green apples
3/4 cup golden raisins
1/2 cup walnuts
2 heads Boston lettuce
1/2 cup low-fat yogurt
1/4 cup mayonnaise
1 tablespoon curry powder
salt and pepper

Remove skin from thighs, place in a medium saucepan, fill with water 2 inches over meat. Place pan over medium-high flame and bring to a gentle simmer. Skim all the scum and fat that comes to the surface, and add onion, celery, carrot, and bay leaf. Simmer for 45 minutes, skimming from time to time. Turn off heat and transfer to a bowl, allow chicken to cool in broth.

Remove meat from thigh bones in large pieces and make sure to remove vein. Dice meat into half-inch cubes. Strain broth and freeze it for future use.

Dice two of the apples in quarter-inch cubes, leaving on skin. Mix with walnuts and raisins. Whisk yogurt, mayonnaise, and curry until smooth. Fold in apple-nut mixture. Fold in chicken and add salt and pepper to taste. Let sit covered in refrigerator.

Remove tough leaves and core from lettuce and wash leaves in large bowl of cold water. Spin dry. Arrange beds of lettuce on four plates. Slice remaining two green apples in half, remove core, and slice halves into quarter-inch slices. Arrange slices on lettuce and distribute chicken salad in mound over the apple slices and lettuce.

## GAZPACHO WITH AVOCADO CREAM

*Cold vegetable soup thick with celery, cucumber, sweet and hot pep-*
*pers, scallions, carrots, and tomato, flavored with extra virgin olive*
*oil, red wine vinegar, and herbs. Served with hearty grain bread.*
*Serves two.*

1 cucumber
1 carrot
2 ribs celery
1 tomato
1 green pepper
1 jalapeño pepper
4 scallions
1/8 cup chopped parsley
1 eight-ounce can V-8 juice
1 eight-ounce can tomato juice
1 teaspoon Worcestershire sauce
1-1/2 tablespoon red wine vinegar
dash hot sauce
salt and fresh ground black pepper
1 ripe avocado
1/2 lime
salt and pepper
extra virgin olive oil

Peel carrot and cucumber. Remove seeds from cucumber
by cutting lengthwise and scooping with a spoon. Cut tomato in half east-west and remove seeds and core at top. Cut
peppers in half and remove seeds, stems, and ribs. Finely dice
peppers and cucumber and set aside in large bowl.

Rough chop carrot, scallion, and celery. Pulse in food processor until finely chopped but not starting to lose liquid, and add to bowl. Repeat with tomato. Add parsley to bowl as well as juices, Worcestershire, vinegar, and hot sauce. Adjust seasoning with salt and pepper. Chill well.

Cut avocado in half, remove pit, and scoop out from skin into processor. Add juice of half a lime and process until smooth. Add salt and pepper to taste.

Ladle soup into chilled bowls and dollop avocado in center. Lace top with a quick swirl of olive oil. Serve with hearty bread.

## TURKEY TABBOULEH

*Bulgur grain mixed with diced turkey breast, tomatoes, olives, scallion, and chopped parsley, finished with lemon and olive oil. Served on a bed of shredded iceberg lettuce. Serves four.*

1 cup bulgur grain
1 cup boiling water
1 teaspoon salt
2 tomatoes
1/2 cup pitted Kalamata olives
1 bunch scallions
2 bunches flat-leaf parsley
1 large lemon
1/4 cup olive oil
salt and pepper
1 lb roast turkey breast, cut into half-inch cubes
1 small head iceberg lettuce, shredded

Place bulgur and salt in a medium bowl, add boiling water, and cover with plastic wrap. Let soak until liquid is absorbed, about 35 minutes.

Cut tomatoes east-west, remove core at top, and chop into quarter-inch pieces. Place in medium bowl and set aside. Trim and clean scallion in cold water and chop, add to tomatoes. Wash parsley in large bowl of cold water, shake or spin dry, and chop, avoiding stems. Slice olives and add to tomatoes with parsley. Dice turkey in half-inch cubes and add to vegetables.

Remove plastic from bowl of bulgur and fluff the grain with a fork. Squeeze lemon juice and add to bulgur with olive oil, continuing to fluff. Add vegetables and turkey by fluffing in, and add salt and fresh-ground pepper to taste. Place lettuce on four plates and spoon tabbouleh over lettuce.

## CLASSIC CLUB BROCCOLI SALAD

*Crisp blanched broccoli tossed with bacon, currants, and smoked almonds. Serves two.*

1 head broccoli
salt
4 slices bacon
4 ounces smoked almonds
1/4 cup currants
1/3 cup mayonnaise
1 tablespoon distilled vinegar
1 tablespoon sugar
salt and fresh-ground black pepper

Fill a large bowl with ice water, set aside. Cut florets off in bite-size pieces. Bring a medium pot of water to a boil and add salt until it has something of an ocean-like taste. Drop broccoli in water and cook 1 minute. Lift out broccoli with slotted spoon and plunge into bowl of ice water. When broccoli is cool, drain and place in colander to dry out.

Cook bacon in skillet or microwave until crisp. Crumble bacon and mix in bowl with smoked almonds and currants.

Whisk mayonnaise, vinegar, and sugar. Fold in broccoli and nut mixture. Add salt and fresh ground pepper to taste.

## ASIAN SHRIMP SALAD

*Shrimp, sweet peppers, scallions, grapes, cilantro, and crushed peanuts dressed with a sweet and sour sauce. Serves four.*

1 lb peeled, raw shrimp
1 teaspoon Chinese five-spice powder
1 teaspoon salt
1/2 tablespoon peanut oil
1 red pepper
1 bunch scallion
1 carrot
1 bunch watercress
1/8 cup chopped cilantro
juice of 1 lime
1 teaspoon fish sauce
1 tablespoon rice vinegar
1 teaspoon sugar
1/2 lb seedless grapes
1/4 cup peanuts, crushed

Heat skillet over medium-high heat and test with water drop for fast sputter. Add peanut oil, sprinkle shrimp with five-spice powder and salt, and sear in skillet on each side until firm and cooked (times vary by size of shrimp, but about 90 seconds each side should do). Set aside cooked shrimp to cool.

Wash scallions and slice on a diagonal in one-inch lengths. Core, seed, and remove ribs from pepper and slice in one-inch lengths. Trim end of watercress, chop in one-inch lengths, wash in cold water and spin dry. Combine all in large bowl.

Whisk lime juice, fish sauce, vinegar, and sugar together. Pour over vegetables and toss. Place mixture on platter, arrange shrimp on top, and sprinkle with crushed peanuts. Garnish with grapes.

## GREEK DINNER SALAD

*Romaine and spinach garnished with cucumbers, tomato, olive, onion, and feta cheese. Topped with marinated chicken breast brushed with an herb vinaigrette. Serves four.*

2 full boneless, skinless chicken breasts
2 lemons
1/2 cup olive oil
1 teaspoon dried oregano
1 small clove garlic, minced
1/4 teaspoon fresh ground pepper
1 teaspoon salt
1 head romaine lettuce
1 bunch leaf spinach
1 cucumber
2 tomatoes
1/2 red onion
1/2 cup Kalamata olives
8 ounces feta cheese

With the fine side of a box grater, grate the yellow part of skin of one lemon. Place in jar or Tupperware with lid. Add juice from lemons, oregano, salt, pepper, garlic, and olive oil. Shake briskly.

Cut chicken breasts along breastbone to separate in two pieces each. Trim off cartilage, fat, and tenders. Place each piece between plastic wrap and pound evenly to about a half-inch thickness. Place pieces in a pan where they do not overlap and pour one-third of dressing over them and turn to coat. Cover with plastic and place in refrigerator.

Trim and clean lettuce and spinach in bowl of cold water. Lift leaves out and repeat washing with fresh, cold water. Chop leaves into three-quarter-inch pieces and spin dry.

Peel and seed cucumber and slice halves into quarter-inch slices. Remove top core of tomatoes and cut eight wedges from each tomato. Slice onion half as thinly as possible.

Pat chicken dry with paper towel and season with salt, pepper, and rub on some olive oil. Place in pan under broiler and cook through, flipping the breasts when halfway done. Remove from oven and brush breasts with some of the vinaigrette.

Toss leaves with remaining vinaigrette and adjust salt and ground pepper. Create a bed of leaves on each plate, arrange four tomato wedges on each and equally distribute the cucumber, onion, olives, and feta cheese. Top with a chicken breast each.

## TUNA NIÇOISE SALAD

*Green beans, tomato, hard-boiled egg, Niçoise olives, and tuna on bibb lettuce, Dijon vinaigrette. Serves two.*

2 eggs
1 tomato
4 ounces French green beans
2 ounces Niçoise olives
1/4 red onion
4 small red or yellow potatoes
1 teaspoon salt
1 six-ounce can tuna packed in olive oil
2 heads bibb lettuce
1 teaspoon Dijon mustard
1/2 clove garlic, minced
juice of one lemon
1 teaspoon sugar
1/4 cup olive oil
pinch dried thyme

Place eggs in small pan, cover with water, and bring to a simmer over medium-high heat. Cover and turn off heat. After 7 minutes, remove eggs and plunge in ice water.

Place potatoes in small pan with water to cover and salt. Bring to a simmer over medium-high heat, and cook until knife can easily penetrate. Cool.

Bring a medium pan of water to a boil with enough salt to make it taste almost like the ocean. Trim beans and cook 2 minutes. Remove with slotted spoon and plunge into ice water. When beans are cool, drain them.

Prepare vinaigrette by combining mustard, sugar, thyme, and garlic in a small bowl with a whisk. Add olive oil, a drop at a time at first to whisk into an emulsion. Gradually add oil in a steady thin stream while continuously whisking. Season with salt and fresh ground pepper.

Trim and wash bibb lettuce and spin dry. Peel eggs and cut in quarters. Cut small potatoes in quarters. Slice onion as thinly as possible. Core and cut tomato into wedges. Place lettuce on platter in a bed and arrange vegetables and eggs around perimiter of the platter. Place drained tuna in center and garnish with olives. Serve vinaigrette on the side.

# Dinner

## SOBA PRIMAVERA

*Japanese buckwheat noodles tossed with sautéed greens, garlic, grape tomato, olives, parmesan cheese and chives. Serves two.*

2 bundles (about 4 ounces) soba noodles
1 tablespoon salt
olive oil
1 bunch kale, trimmed and washed
1 portabella mushroom, wiped clean and diced
1/2 cup grape tomatoes, halved
1/2 cup olives, sliced
1 clove minced garlic
1 peeled and thinly sliced shallot
3-ounce piece parmesan, grated
1/3 bunch chives, chopped

Bring a medium pot of water to a boil with the salt. Add soba and cook according to time on package. Reserve 1 cup of cooking water, drain noodles.

Heat large sauté pan over medium-high heat, add about 1 tablespoon of olive oil and the mushroom. Allow to cook until released liquid has dried and add garlic, shallot, olives, and tomatoes. Season with salt and pepper and cook another 2 minutes. Put vegetables in a bowl, wipe pan with paper towel, add a half tablespoon of olive oil and heat until almost smoking. Add kale and sauté about 30 seconds to coat with oil and add about a third cup of reserved noodle water to pan and cover with a lid. Cook down until kale is tender, stirring occasionally, about 3 minutes. Add vegetables, noodles, and parmesan cheese and toss all ingredients together. Add a bit more reserved noodle water if dish starts to get dry. Divide between two plates and sprinkle chives on top.

## PESTO BLUEFISH

*Basil-crusted bluefish with broccoli and tomato sautéed with shallot and white wine. Serves two.*

12 ounce bluefish fillet
2 slices white bread, crust removed and diced
1 bunch basil, cleaned and chopped
1/4 cup pine nuts
2 ounces parmesan cheese, grated
1 tablespoon olive oil
salt and pepper
olive oil
1 bunch broccoli, florets removed in bite-size pieces
1 tomato, seeded and chopped
juice of 1 lemon
1 shallot, peeled and minced
1 garlic clove, thinly sliced
1/4 cup dry white wine
1/2 tablespoon butter

Set oven to 400°F. Place a medium pot of water over a high flame with enough salt so it almost tastes like the ocean.

In a food processor, grind the bread to a fine crumb and set aside in a bowl. Next process the basil and pine nuts in pulses to break them down, stopping every three or four pulses to wipe down the sides with a spatula. When the mixture becomes fairly smooth, add parmesan and blend in. Next add olive oil in a steady stream while machine is running. Fold mixture into crumbs and season with salt and pepper to taste.

Cut fillet in two pieces. With the back of a spoon, smear pesto on surface of the fish in an even quarter-inch layer. Place fillets in a buttered pan crust side up and add a few tablespoons of water. Bake in oven until cooked through and top is slightly brown, about 12 minutes.

While fish cooks, heat a large sauté pan over medium-high heat. Add broccoli to boiling salted water. Pour about a half tablespoon of oil in sauté pan along with garlic and shallot, stirring to avoid burning for about 1 minute. Add tomatoes and cook another minute. Add wine and allow liquid to reduce about 1 minute. Remove broccoli from boiling water with a slotted spoon and place broccoli directly in sauté pan with tomato mixture. Add lemon juice and butter, reduce heat to medium, and swirl around until butter mounts sauce—do not overheat or butter will break. Remove pan from heat and adjust seasoning with salt and fresh ground pepper. Divide mixture between two plates and top with fish.

## MEDITERRANEAN SALMON

*Broiled salmon with spicy ratatouille (stewed eggplant, yellow and green squash, and red peppers).*

1 twelve-ounce center salmon filet
2 tablespoons butter
1/2 tablespoon chopped fresh parsley
1/2 teaspoon fresh lemon zest
salt and fresh ground pepper
olive oil
1 small to medium yellow squash
1 small to medium zucchini
1 red pepper
1 medium eggplant
1/2 red onion
2 cloves garlic, minced
1 pinch red pepper flakes
1 pinch dried thyme
2 tablespoons tomato paste

Cut squash, zucchini, and eggplant in half-inch cubes by cutting along the side of the vegetable a third-inch deep to produce "sheets," and cut each sheet into cubes. Discard the seedy cores. Dice onion in half-inch pieces.

Mix butter with parsley and lemon. Add salt and pepper to taste.

Heat a medium sauté pan over medium-high heat with about a quarter tablespoon of olive oil and add yellow squash. Season squash with salt and pepper and lower flame to medium, making sure squash is cooked through but not mushy. Set aside in a medium saucepan. Repeat with zucchini, eggplant, and red pepper. Sauté onion until translucent over medium heat and add pepper flakes, thyme, and garlic. Cook 1 minute and add tomato paste, mixing around so the paste comes into as much contact with sauté pan surface as possible. Fold this into the rest of the vegetables in the saucepan and set aside over very low flame. Adjust seasoning with salt and fresh ground pepper.

Heat broiler on high. Cut fish in two, season with salt and fresh ground pepper, and place on foil-lined sheet pan rubbed with a little olive oil. Place pan a few inches from broiler and cook through on one side, allowing to brown a little on top.

Distribute ratatouille between two plates and place salmon on top. Top each piece of hot fish with compound butter and allow to melt over fish.

## MACKEREL ESCABECHE

*Spanish mackerel sautéed and then marinated in a mixture of onions, peppers, and sherry vinegar. Serve with spinach and wheat berry sauté. Serves two.*

olive oil
12-ounce mackerel filet
flour for dredging
1 small red onion, thinly sliced
1 yellow or red pepper, sliced
3/4 cup sherry vinegar
1/2 cup water
2 cloves garlic, sliced thin
1/2 tablespoon sugar
pinch red pepper flakes
1/2 cup wheat berries
1 cup water
2 teaspoons salt
2 bunch leafy spinach, trimmed and washed
salt and fresh ground pepper

Heat wheat berries, salt, and water in a small saucepan over medium-high heat. When water starts to simmer, cover with lid and reduce heat to lowest setting. Wheat berries should cook in about 35 minutes—test and add more water if necessary.

Heat medium skillet over medium-high heat. Cut fish in two even pieces, season with salt and pepper, and dredge in flour. Add a half tablespoon of olive oil and sauté fish on both sides until cooked through. Remove fish from pan and set aside in pie pan or similar dish.

Put a half tablespoon of olive oil in pan along with onions and peppers. Cook over medium flame for about 3 minutes or until starting to soften. Drain excess oil from pan and add garlic and pepper flakes. Stir over medium-high flame 30 seconds, deglaze with water and vinegar, and add sugar. When sugar dissolves and onions are soft, pour over fish. Let sit.

Wipe sauté pan with a paper towel and return to high flame. Add about half a tablespoon olive oil and heat to nearly smoking. Add spinach and a generous pinch of salt and sauté. When spinach is wilted, add cooked wheat berries. Spinach is finished when tender, about 1 minute more. Divide among two plates. Serve with marinated fish.

## SPICY GRILLED SHRIMP AND QUINOA

*Shrimp dusted with spice and grilled, served with quinoa salad with avocado, cucumber, cilantro, and lime. Serves two.*

3/4 lb large shrimp, peeled
1 teaspoon cumin
1 teaspoon salt
1/2 teaspoon paprika
1/4 teaspoon ground black pepper
1/2 cup quinoa
1-1/2 cupc water
1/2 teaspoon salt
1 cucumber
3 scallions
1 avocado
1 lime
1/4 cup chopped cilantro
1 tablespoon olive oil
salt and pepper
romaine lettuce
lime wedges

Mix cumin, salt, paprika, and black pepper. Rinse quinoa with cold water. Place in pan with one and a half cups water and salt. Bring to a boil, cover, and reduce heat to low. Quinoa will be ready in 12–15 minutes. Remove lid and fluff with a fork.

Peel cucumber, slice in half lengthwise, and remove seeds with a spoon. Dice halves into quarter-inch pieces.

Clean scallions and slice thin crosswise, use green and white parts but discard roots at base.

Cut avocado in half around pit. Pull apart, remove pit, and separate skin from halves with a large spoon. Dice avocado halves into quarter-inch pieces and immediately toss with lime juice. Add to cooked quinoa along with cucumber, scallions, and cilantro. Fluff in olive oil and add salt and fresh ground pepper to taste.

Heat a large skillet over medium–high heat, add about half a tablespoon olive oil and swirl it around in the pan. Toss shrimp with spice mixture and add shrimp to pan, one at a time, gently pressing shrimp on pan surface. Allow to sear about 90 seconds or until color, flip, and finish cooking. Line two plates with romaine, place half quinoa mixture in center of each plate, and arrange shrimp around the salad. Serve with additional lime wedges.

## STEAK WITH CREAM SPINACH AND MILLET CROQUETTES

*Your favorite steak simply prepared and combined with a healthy dose of spinach and millet. Serves four.*

Steak of your choice, prepared your desired method
4 bunches curly spinach, washed and trimmed
1/4 cup cream
salt and pepper
1/2 cup millet
2 cups water
3 scallions, washed and chopped
1 clove garlic, minced
1 red pepper, small dice
1 teaspoon Worcestershire
1 dash Tabasco
1 egg, scrambled
2 ounces parmesan, grated
1/4 cup all-purpose flour
olive oil

Fill large pot with water and bring to a boil. Add enough salt so water tastes almost like the ocean. Add spinach and cook until tender, about 2 minutes after water returns to a boil. Remove spinach and plunge into cold water. Squeeze spinach dry and put in processor. Pulse until spinach breaks up evenly, scraping down sides. When fairly uniform, run processor continuously and add cream in a steady stream. Add salt and fresh ground pepper to taste.

Bring millet and water to a boil, cover, and simmer until liquid is gone, about 30 minutes. Set aside and let rest.

In a sauté pan, add about half a tablespoon of olive oil and sauté pepper with scallion until soft. Add garlic and cook 30 seconds more. Fluff millet with fork, add scallion mixture, Tabasco, Worcestershire sauce, egg, parmesan, and flour and combine. Add salt and pepper to taste. Form mixture into golfball-size pieces and flatten into disks. Heat skillet with olive oil and cook until brown. Flip and put in oven 12 minutes or until cooked through. Serve on platter with reheated cream spinach and steaks.

## SOUTHERN STUFFED PORK CHOPS AND RED FLANNEL HASH

*Pork chops stuffed with Swiss chard and served with hash made from sweet potato, beets and bacon. Serves four.*

4 six-ounce pork chops
1 bunch Swiss chard
olive oil
2 red onions chopped, divided in two
1 clove garlic, minced
2 tablespoons white vinegar
dash of Tabasco sauce
1/4 cup cream
2 tablespoons bulgur
3/4 cups white wine
1/2 tablespoon corn starch
1 tablespoon water
2 sweet potatoes
2 medium beets
4 slices bacon
1/4 cup sour cream
2 tablespoon Dijon mustard
1/8 cup chopped parsley
salt and pepper

Set oven to 375°F. Wash and dry beets and sweet potatoes, prick all around with a knife, rub with olive oil, season with salt and pepper, and wrap in foil. Place in oven and cook until knife is easily inserted, about an hour.

Set a medium pan filled with water over high flame and bring to a boil. Trim and wash Swiss chard in large bowl of cold water, shake dry, and chop into two-inch pieces. Add enough salt to boiling water so it almost tastes like the ocean and add Swiss chard. Cook until tender, about 4–6 minutes. Drain chard from pot and plunge into ice-cold water.

Place a sauté pan over medium heat, add a half tablespoon olive oil and halve the onions. Cook until onions are translucent. Add garlic and turn up heat to medium high. Cook garlic about 30 seconds, stirring, and add Swiss chard. Cook another minute and add vinegar. After vinegar reduces (about a minute) add cream and bulgur. Stir until thickened, and set aside to cool.

With a small knife, cut into center of the side opposite the bone of each pork chop. Once knife is inserted, pivot it carefully from side to side, avoiding breaking all the way through, to make a pocket. Stuff each pocket with one-quarter of the stuffing and close pocket with toothpicks.

Heat a sauté pan just large enough for the chops with a half tablespoon olive oil. Season chops with salt and pepper and sear on each side. Remove chops from pan and deglaze with wine. Reduce by half, turn off heat, return chops to pan, and cover pan with foil. Place in oven and cook until done, being careful not to dry out chops (begin checking after 20 minutes).

Peel cooled sweet potatoes and beets. Dice into quarter-inch pieces and mix in with parsley, mustard, and sour cream. Add salt and pepper to taste. Heat bacon in skillet until crisp and crumble bacon in with mixture. Pour mixture into pan with bacon drippings, spread evenly and cook over medium-high heat until crisp. Flip and crisp on other side.

Remove chops from pan and return to medium-high flame. Combine cornstarch with water to make a slurry and whisk into juices to make a gravy. Gravy will thicken when it reaches a boil. Cook another minute and adjust seasoning.

Divide hash among four plates, give each a chop, and serve with gravy.

# References

## CHAPTER 1
## PAIN-FREE LIVING: UNDERSTANDING
## INFLAMMATORY BALANCE

Adam O., Beringer C., Kless T., Lemmen C., Adam A., Wiseman M., Adam P., Klimmek R., Forth W. "Anti-inflammatory effects of a low arachidonic acid diet and fish oil in patients with rheumatoid arthritis. *Rheumatol Int.* 2003 Jan;23(1):27–36.

Belch JJ, Hill A. Evening primrose oil and borage oil in rheumatologic conditions. *Am J Clin Nutr.* 2000 Jan;71(1 Suppl):352S–6S.

Buchanan WW, Kean WF, Rooney PJ. Some metabolic aspects of arthritis. *S Afr Med J.* 1982 Mar 27;61(13):467–71.

Calder PC. Dietary modification of inflammation with lipids. *Proc Nutr Soc.* 2002 Aug;61(3):345–58.

Calder PC. n-3 polyunsaturated fatty acids and cytokine production in health and disease. *Ann Nutr Metab.* 1997;41(4):203–34.

Calder PC. Polyunsaturated fatty acids, inflammation, and immunity. *Lipids.* 2001 Sep;36(9):1007–24.

Chang SY, Howden CW. Is no NSAID a good NSAID? Approaches to NSAID-associated upper gastrointestinal disease. *Curr Gastroenterol Rep.* 2004 Dec;6(6):447–53.

Chiolero A, Maillard MP, Burnier M. Cardiovascular hazard of selective COX-2 inhibitors: myth or reality? *Expert Opin Drug Saf.* 2002 May;1(1):45–52.

Cleland LG, Hill CL, James MJ. Diet and arthritis. *Baillieres Clin Rheumatol.* 1995 Nov;9(4):771–85.

Danao-Camara TC, Shintani TT. The dietary treatment of inflammatory arthritis: case reports and review of the literature. *Hawaii Med J.* 1999 May;58(5):126–31.

Fortun PJ, Hawkey CJ. Life after Vioxx: the clinical implications. *Hosp Med.* 2005 May;66(5):264–7.

Gil A. Polyunsaturated fatty acids and inflammatory diseases. *Biomed Pharmacother.* 2002 Oct;56(8):388–96.

Grimble RF, Tappia PS. Modulation of pro-inflammatory cytokine biology by unsaturated fatty acids. *Z Ernahrungswiss.* 1998;37 Suppl 1:57–65.

Halliwell B. Effect of diet on cancer development: is oxidative DNA damage a biomarker? *Free Radic Biol Med.* 2002 May 15;32(10):968–74.

Hawkey CJ. Cyclooxygenase inhibition: between the devil and the deep blue sea. *Gut.* 2002 May;50 Suppl 3:III 25–30.

Hochberg MC. COX-2 selective inhibitors in the treatment of arthritis: a rheumatologist perspective. *Curr Top Med Chem.* 2005;5(5):443–8.

Hochberg MC. Treatment of rheumatoid arthritis and osteoarthritis with COX-2-selective inhibitors: a managed care perspective. *Am J Manag Care.* 2002 Nov;8(17 Suppl):S502–17.

Howes LG, Krum H. Selective cyclo-oxygenase-2 inhibitors and myocardial infarction: how strong is the link? *Drug Saf.* 2002;25(12):829–35.

James MJ, Gibson RA, Cleland LG. Dietary polyunsaturated fatty acids and inflammatory mediator production. *Am J Clin Nutr.* 2000 Jan;71(1 Suppl):343S–8S.

Kremer JM. n-3 fatty acid supplements in rheumatoid arthritis. *Am J Clin Nutr.* 2000 Jan;71(1 Suppl):349S–51S.

Mardini IA, FitzGerald GA. Selective inhibitors of cyclooxygenase-2: a growing class of anti-inflammatory drugs. *Mol Interv.* 2001 Apr;1(1):30–8.

Mukherjee D. Selective cyclooxygenase-2 (COX-2) inhibitors and potential risk of cardiovascular events. *Biochem Pharmacol.* 2002 Mar 1;63(5):817–21.

Oviedo JA, Wolfe MM. Gastroprotection by coxibs: what do the Celecoxib Long-Term Arthritis Safety Study and the Vioxx Gastrointestinal Outcomes Research Trial tell us? *Rheum Dis Clin North Am.* 2003 Nov;29(4):769–88.

Pattison DJ, Symmons DP, Young A. Does diet have a role in the aetiology of rheumatoid arthritis? *Proc Nutr Soc.* 2004 Feb;63(1):137–43.

Ray WA, MacDonald TM, Solomon DH, Graham DJ, Avorn J. COX-2 selective non-steroidal anti-inflammatory drugs and cardiovascular disease. *Pharmacoepidemiol Drug Saf.* 2003 Jan-Feb;12(1):67–70.

Sanders HJ. Arthritis and drugs; the ongoing quest to reveal its causes. II. IMS *Ind Med Surg.* 1969 Sep;38(9):290–308.

Simopoulos AP. Omega-3 fatty acids in inflammation and autoimmune diseases. *J Am Coll Nutr.* 2002 Dec;21(6):495–505.

Simopoulos AP. The importance of the ratio of omega-6/omega-3 essential fatty acids. *Biomed Pharmacother.* 2002 Oct;56(8):365–79.

Spiegel BM, Targownik L, Dulai GS, Gralnek IM. The cost-effectiveness of cyclooxygenase-2 selective inhibitors in the management of chronic arthritis. *Ann Intern Med.* 2003 May 20;138(10):795–806.

Strand V, Hochberg MC. The risk of cardiovascular thrombotic events with selective cyclooxygenase-2 inhibitors. *Arthritis Rheum.* 2002 Aug;47(4):349–55.

Wright JM. The double-edged sword of COX-2 selective NSAIDs. *CMAJ.* 2002 Nov 12;167(10):1131–7.

# CHAPTER 2
## CONNECTIVE TISSUE: THE FOUNDATION ON WHICH WE'RE BUILT

Bartecchi CE. Fibromyalgia and complementary and alternative medicine. *Mayo Clin Proc.* 2005 Jun;80(6):826.

Bora FW Jr, Miller G. Joint physiology, cartilage metabolism, and the etiology of osteoarthritis. *Hand Clin.* 1987 Aug;3(3):325–36.

Bullough PG. The role of joint architecture in the etiology of arthritis. *Osteoarthritis Cartilage.* 2004;12 Suppl A:S2–9.

Cusack S, Cashman KD. Impact of genetic variation on metabolic response of bone to diet. *Proc Nutr Soc.* 2003 Nov;62(4):901–12.

Davies JH, Evans BA, Gregory JW. Bone mass acquisition in healthy children. *Arch Dis Child.* 2005 Apr;90(4):373–8.

Fries E, Hesse J, Hellhammer J, Hellhammer DH. A new view on hypocortisolism. *Psychoneuroendocrinology.* 2005 Nov;30(10):1010–6.

Goggs R, Vaughan-Thomas A, Clegg PD, Carter SD, Innes JF, Mobasheri A, Shakibaei M, Schwab W, Bondy CA. Nutraceutical therapies for degenerative joint diseases: a critical review. *Crit Rev Food Sci Nutr.* 2005;45(3):145–64.

Hulth A. Does osteoarthrosis depend on growth of the mineralized layer of cartilage? *Clin Orthop Relat Res.* 1993 Feb;(287):19–24.

Imhof H, Breitenseher M, Kainberger F, Rand T, Trattnig S. Importance of subchondral bone to articular cartilage in health and disease. *Top Magn Reson Imaging.* 1999 Jun;10(3):180–92.

Krane SM, Goldring MB. Clinical implications of cartilage metabolism in arthritis. *Eur J Rheumatol Inflamm.* 1990;10(1):4–9.

Lane JM, Russell L, Khan SN. Osteoporosis. *Clin Orthop Relat Res.* 2000 Mar;(372):139–50.

Lane JM. Osteoporosis. Medical prevention and treatment. *Spine.* 1997 Dec 15;22(24 Suppl):32S–37S.

Luedtke CA, Thompson JM, Postier JA, Neubauer BL, Drach S, Newell L. A description of a brief multidisciplinary treatment program for fibromyalgia. *Pain Manag Nurs.* 2005 Jun;6(2):76–80.

Ralston SH. What determines peak bone mass and bone loss? *Baillieres Clin Rheumatol.* 1997 Aug;11(3):479–94.

Smythe HA. Incarnations of fibromyalgia. *J Rheumatol.* 2005 Aug;32(8):1422–5.

# CHAPTER 3
# THE GRAYING OF AMERICA: AGING AS A BALANCE BETWEEN CONNECTIVE TISSUE BREAKDOWN AND REPAIR

Aigner T, Kurz B, Fukui N, Sandell L. Roles of chondrocytes in the pathogenesis of osteoarthritis. *Curr Opin Rheumatol.* 2002 Sep;14(5):578–84.

Carbone LD, Tylavsky FA, Cauley JA, Harris TB, Lang TF, Bauer DC, Barrow KD, Kritchevsky SB. Association between bone mineral density and the use of nonsteroidal anti-inflammatory drugs and aspirin: impact of cyclooxygenase selectivity. *J Bone Miner Res.* 2003 Oct;18(10):1795–802.

Corvol MT. The chondrocyte: from cell aging to osteoarthritis. *Joint Bone Spine.* 2000;67(6):557–60.

DeGroot J, Verzijl N, Bank RA, Lafeber FP, Bijlsma JW, TeKoppele JM. Age-related decrease in proteoglycan synthesis of human articular chondrocytes: the role of nonenzymatic glycation. *Arthritis Rheum.* 1999 May;42(5):1003–9.

DeGroot J, Verzijl N, Wenting-Van Wijk MJ, Bank RA, Lafeber FP, Bijlsma JW, TeKoppele JM. Age-related decrease in susceptibility of human articular cartilage to matrix metalloproteinase-mediated degradation: the role of advanced glycation end products. *Arthritis Rheum.* 2001 Nov;44(11):2562–71.

Dequeker J, Aerssens J, Luyten FP. Osteoarthritis and osteoporosis: clinical and research evidence of inverse relationship. *Aging Clin Exp Res.* 2003 Oct;15(5):426–39.

Dozin B, Malpeli M, Camardella L, Cancedda R, Pietrangelo A. Response of young, aged and osteoarthritic human articular chondrocytes to inflammatory cytokines: molecular and cellular aspects. *Matrix Biol.* 2002 Aug;21(5):449–59.

Helminen HJ, Hyttinen MM, Lammi MJ, Arokoski JP, Lapvetelainen T, Jurvelin J, Kiviranta I, Tammi MI. Regular joint loading in youth assists in the establishment and strengthening of the collagen network of articular cartilage and contributes to the prevention of osteoarthrosis later in life: a hypothesis. *J Bone Miner Metab.* 2000;18(5):245–57.

Holick MF. Sunlight and vitamin D for bone health and prevention of autoimmune diseases, cancers, and cardiovascular disease. *Am J Clin Nutr.* 2004 Dec;80(6 Suppl):1678S–88S.

Hollander AP, Pidoux I, Reiner A, Rorabeck C, Bourne R, Poole AR. Damage to type II collagen in aging and osteoarthritis starts at the articular surface, originates around chondrocytes, and extends into the cartilage with progressive degeneration. *J Clin Invest.* 1995 Dec;96(6):2859–69.

Ishiguro N, Kojima T, Poole AR. Mechanism of cartilage destruction in osteoarthritis. *Nagoya J Med Sci.* 2002 Nov;65(3–4):73–84.

Loeser RF Jr. Aging cartilage and osteoarthritis—-what"s the link? *Sci Aging Knowledge Environ.* 2004 Jul 21;2004(29):pe31.

Loeser RF, Yammani RR, Carlson CS, Chen H, Cole A, Im HJ, Bursch LS, Yan SD. Articular chondrocytes express the receptor for advanced glycation end products: Potential role in osteoarthritis. *Arthritis Rheum.* 2005 Aug;52(8):2376–85.

Martin JA, Brown T, Heiner A, Buckwalter JA. Post-traumatic osteoarthritis: the role of accelerated chondrocyte senescence. *Biorheology.* 2004;41(3-4):479–91.

Martin JA, Buckwalter JA. Aging, articular cartilage chondrocyte senescence and osteoarthritis. *Biogerontology.* 2002;3(5):257–64.

Martin JA, Buckwalter JA. Roles of articular cartilage aging and chondrocyte senescence in the pathogenesis of osteoarthritis. *Iowa Orthop J.* 2001;21:1–7.

Martin JA, Buckwalter JA. The role of chondrocyte senescence in the pathogenesis of osteoarthritis and in limiting cartilage repair. *J Bone Joint Surg Am.* 2003;85–A Suppl 2:106–10.

Martin JA, Klingelhutz AJ, Moussavi-Harami F, Buckwalter JA. Effects of oxidative damage and telomerase activity on human articular cartilage chondrocyte senescence. *J Gerontol A Biol Sci Med Sci.* 2004 Apr;59 (4):324–37.

Min BH, Kim HJ, Lim H, Park CS, Park SR. Effects of ageing and arthritic disease on nitric oxide production by human articular chondrocytes. *Exp Mol Med.* 2001 Dec 31;33(4):299–302.

Poole AR, Nelson F, Dahlberg L, Tchetina E, Kobayashi M, Yasuda T, Laverty S, Squires G, Kojima T, Wu W, Billinghurst RC. Proteolysis of the collagen fibril in osteoarthritis. *Biochem Soc Symp.* 2003;(70):115–23.

Price JS, Waters JG, Darrah C, Pennington C, Edwards DR, Donell ST, Clark IM. The role of chondrocyte senescence in osteoarthritis. *Aging Cell.* 2002 Oct;1(1):57–65.

Rutsch F, Terkeltaub R. Deficiencies of physiologic calcification inhibitors and low-grade inflammation in arterial calcification: lessons for cartilage calcification. *Joint Bone Spine.* 2005 Mar;72(2):110–8.

Ulrich-Vinther M, Maloney MD, Schwarz EM, Rosier R, O'Keefe RJ.

Articular cartilage biology. *J Am Acad Orthop Surg.* 2003 Nov–Dec;11 (6):421–30.

Verzijl N, Bank RA, TeKoppele JM, DeGroot J. AGEing and osteoarthritis: a different perspective. *Curr Opin Rheumatol.* 2003 Sep;15(5):616–22.

Verzijl N, DeGroot J, Ben ZC, Brau-Benjamin O, Maroudas A, Bank RA, Mizrahi J, Schalkwijk CG, Thorpe SR, Baynes JW, Bijlsma JW, Lafeber FP, TeKoppele JM. Crosslinking by advanced glycation end products increases the stiffness of the collagen network in human articular cartilage: a possible mechanism through which age is a risk factor for osteoarthritis. *Arthritis Rheum.* 2002 Jan;46(1):114–23.

# CHAPTER 4
## EATING FOR FLEXIBILITY: SUPPORTING INJURY REPAIR WITH NUTRITION

Araujo V, Arnal C, Boronat M, Ruiz E, Dominguez C. Oxidant-antioxidant imbalance in blood of children with juvenile rheumatoid arthritis. *Biofactors.* 1998;8(1–2):155–9.

Babraj JA, Smith K, Cuthbertson DJ, Rickhuss P, Dorling JS, Rennie MJ. Human bone collagen synthesis is a rapid, nutritionally modulated process. *J Bone Miner Res.* 2005 Jun;20(6):930–7. Epub 2005 Feb 14.

Ballard TL, Clapper JA, Specker BL, Binkley TL, Vukovich MD. Effect of protein supplementation during a 6-mo strength and conditioning program on insulin-like growth factor I and markers of bone turnover in young adults. *Am J Clin Nutr.* 2005 Jun;81(6):1442–8.

Basta G, Lazzerini G, Massaro M, Simoncini T, Tanganelli P, Fu C, Kislinger T, Stern DM, Schmidt AM, De Caterina R. Advanced glycation end products activate endothelium through signal-transduction receptor RAGE: a mechanism for amplification of inflammatory responses. *Circulation.* 2002 Feb 19;105(7):816–22.

Frey J. Collagen, ageing and nutrition. *Clin Chem Lab Med.* 2004 Jan;42(1):9–12.

Ginty F, Cavadini C, Michaud PA, Burckhardt P, Baumgartner M, Mishra GD, Barclay DV. Effects of usual nutrient intake and vitamin D status on markers of bone turnover in Swiss adolescents. *Eur J Clin Nutr.* 2004 Sep;58(9):1257–65.

Hajizadeh S, DeGroot J, TeKoppele JM, Tarkowski A, Collins LV. Extracellular mitochondrial DNA and oxidatively damaged DNA in synovial fluid of patients with rheumatoid arthritis. *Arthritis Res Ther.* 2003; 5(5):R234–40.

Heaney RP, McCarron DA, Dawson-Hughes B, Oparil S, Berga SL, Stern JS, Barr SI, Rosen CJ. Dietary changes favorably affect bone remodeling in older adults. *J Am Diet Assoc.* 1999 Oct;99(10):1228–33.

Heer M, Baecker N, Mika C, Boese A, Gerzer R. Immobilization induces a very rapid increase in osteoclast activity. *Acta Astronaut.* 2005 Jul;57(1):31–6.

Henrotin YE, Bruckner P, Pujol JP. The role of reactive oxygen species in homeostasis and degradation of cartilage. *Osteoarthritis Cartilage.* 2003 Oct;11(10):747–55.

Jira W, Spiteller G, Richter A. Increased levels of lipid oxidation products in low density lipoproteins of patients suffering from rheumatoid arthritis. *Chem Phys Lipids.* 1997 May 30;87(1):81–9.

Kalkwarf HJ, Khoury JC, Bean J, Elliot JG. Vitamin K, bone turnover, and bone mass in girls. *Am J Clin Nutr.* 2004 Oct;80(4):1075–80.

Khan M, Pelengaris S, Cooper M, Smith C, Evan G, Betteridge J. Oxidised lipoproteins may promote inflammation through the selective delay of engulfment but not binding of apoptotic cells by macrophages. *Atherosclerosis.* 2003 Nov;171(1):21–9.

Lansdown AB. Nutrition 1: a vital consideration in the management of skin wounds. *Br J Nurs.* 2004 Oct 28–Nov 10;13(19):S22–8.

Lin PH, Ginty F, Appel LJ, Aickin M, Bohannon A, Garnero P, Barclay D, Svetkey LP. The DASH diet and sodium reduction improve markers of bone turnover and calcium metabolism in adults. *J Nutr.* 2003 Oct;133 (10):3130–6.

Mantle D, Wilkins RM, Preedy V. A novel therapeutic strategy for Ehlers-Danlos syndrome based on nutritional supplements. *Med Hypotheses.* 2005;64(2):279–83.

Paredes S, Girona J, Hurt-Camejo E, Vallve JC, Olive S, Heras M, Benito P, Masana L. Antioxidant vitamins and lipid peroxidation in patients with rheumatoid arthritis: association with inflammatory markers. *J Rheumatol.* 2002 Nov;29(11):2271–7.

Russell L. The importance of patients' nutritional status in wound healing. *Br J Nurs.* 2001 Mar;10(6 Suppl):S42, S44–9.

Shackelford LC, LeBlanc AD, Driscoll TB, Evans HJ, Rianon NJ, Smith SM, Spector E, Feeback DL, Lai D. Resistance exercise as a countermeasure to disuse-induced bone loss. *J Appl Physiol.* 2004 Jul;97(1):119–29.

Whitehouse MW. Some chemical aspects of inflammation: a brief overview. *Aust N Z J Med.* 1978;8 Suppl 1:89–93.

Winyard PG, Blake DR. Antioxidants, redox-regulated transcription factors, and inflammation. *Adv Pharmacol.* 1997;38:403–21.

Zanker CL, Cooke CB. Energy balance, bone turnover, and skeletal health in physically active individuals. *Med Sci Sports Exerc.* 2004 Aug;36(8):1372–81.

# CHAPTER 5
# NATURAL DIETARY SUPPLEMENTS AND SUPPORTING NUTRIENTS: GIVING TISSUE REPAIR A HELPING HAND

Adami S, Bufalino L, Cervetti R, Di Marco C, Di Munno O, Fantasia L, Isaia GC, Serni U, Vecchiet L, Passeri M. Ipriflavone prevents radial bone loss in postmenopausal women with low bone mass over 2 years. *Osteoporos Int.* 1997;7(2):119–25.

Agerup B, Berg P, Akermark C. Non-animal stabilized hyaluronic acid: a new formulation for the treatment of osteoarthritis. *BioDrugs.* 2005;19(1):23–30.

Aggarwal BB, Shishodia S. Suppression of the nuclear factor-kappaB activation pathway by spice-derived phytochemicals: reasoning for seasoning. *Ann N Y Acad Sci.* 2004 Dec;1030:434–41.

Agnusdei D, Bufalino L. Efficacy of ipriflavone in established osteoporosis and long-term safety. *Calcif Tissue Int.* 1997;61 Suppl 1:S23–7.

Agnusdei D, Crepaldi G, Isaia G, Mazzuoli G, Ortolani S, Passeri M, Bufalino L, Gennari C. A double blind, placebo-controlled trial of ipriflavone for prevention of postmenopausal spinal bone loss. *Calcif Tissue Int.* 1997 Aug;61(2):142–7.

Alexandersen P, Toussaint A, Christiansen C, Devogelaer JP, Roux C, Fechtenbaum J, Gennari C, Reginster JY; Ipriflavone Multicenter European Fracture Study. Ipriflavone in the treatment of postmenopausal osteoporosis: a randomized controlled trial. *JAMA.* 2001 Mar 21;285(11):1482–8.

Angermann P. Avocado/soybean unsaponifiables in the treatment of knee and hip osteoarthritis. *Ugeskr Laeger.* 2005 Aug 15;167(33):3023–5.

Appelboom T, Schuermans J, Verbruggen G, Henrotin Y, Reginster JY. Symptoms modifying effect of avocado/soybean unsaponifiables (ASU) in knee osteoarthritis. A double blind, prospective, placebo-controlled study. *Scand J Rheumatol.* 2001;30(4):242–7.

Ariyoshi W, Takahashi T, Kanno T, Ichimiya H, Takano H, Koseki T, Nishihara T. Mechanisms involved in enhancement of osteoclast formation and function by low molecular weight hyaluronic acid. *J Biol Chem.* 2005 May 13;280(19):18967–72.

Arora RB, Kapoor V, Basu N, Jain AP. Anti-inflammatory studies on Curcuma longa (turmeric). *Indian J Med Res.* 1971 Aug;59(8):1289–95.

Arora S, Kaur K, Kaur S. Indian medicinal plants as a reservoir of protective phytochemicals. *Teratog Carcinog Mutagen.* 2003;Suppl 1:295–300.

Baker CL Jr, Ferguson CM. Future treatment of osteoarthritis. *Orthopedics.* 2005 Feb;28(2 Suppl):s227–34.

Bassleer CT, Franchimont PP, Henrotin YE, Franchimont NM, Geenen VG, Reginster JY. Effects of ipriflavone and its metabolites on human articular chondrocytes cultivated in clusters. *Osteoarthritis Cartilage.* 1996 Mar;4(1):1–8.

Bliddal H, Rosetzsky A, Schlichting P, Weidner MS, Andersen LA, Ibfelt HH, Christensen K, Jensen ON, Barslev J. A randomized, placebo-controlled, cross-over study of ginger extracts and ibuprofen in osteoarthritis. *Osteoarthritis Cartilage.* 2000 Jan;8(1):9–12.

Boumediene K, Felisaz N, Bogdanowicz P, Galera P, Guillou GB, Pujol JP. Avocado/soya unsaponifiables enhance the expression of transforming growth factor beta1 and beta2 in cultured articular chondrocytes. *Arthritis Rheum.* 1999 Jan;42(1):148–56.

Butenko IG, Gladtchenko SV, Galushko SV. Anti-inflammatory properties and inhibition of leukotriene C4 biosynthesis in vitro by flavonoid baicalein from Scutellaria baicalensis georgy roots. *Agents Actions.* 1993;39 Spec No:C49-51.

Cake MA, Read RA, Guillou B, Ghosh P. Modification of articular cartilage and subchondral bone pathology in an ovine meniscectomy model of osteoarthritis by avocado and soya unsaponifiables (ASU). *Osteoarthritis Cartilage.* 2000 Nov;8(6):404–11.

Cha YY, Lee EO, Lee HJ, Park YD, Ko SG, Kim DH, Kim HM, Kang IC, Kim SH. Methylene chloride fraction of Scutellaria barbata induces apoptosis in human U937 leukemia cells via the mitochondrial signaling pathway. *Clin Chim Acta.* 2004 Oct;348(1-2):41–8.

Chan MM, Ho CT, Huang HI. Effects of three dietary phytochemicals from tea, rosemary and turmeric on inflammation-induced nitrite production. *Cancer Lett.* 1995 Sep 4;96(1):23–9.

Chang ST, Wu JH, Wang SY, Kang PL, Yang NS, Shyur LF. Antioxidant activity of extracts from Acacia confusa bark and heartwood. *J Agric Food Chem.* 2001 Jul;49(7):3420–4.

Chaudhari PN, Hatwalne VG. Effect of Acacia catechu on niacin, ascorbic acid and riboflavin status in rats. *J Vitaminol (Kyoto).* 1970 Jun 10;17(2):105–7.

Chi YS, Kim HP. Suppression of cyclooxygenase-2 expression of skin fibroblasts by wogonin, a plant flavone from Scutellaria radix. *Prostaglandins Leukot Essent Fatty Acids.* 2005 Jan;72(1):59–66.

Chi YS, Lim H, Park H, Kim HP. Effects of wogonin, a plant flavone from Scutellaria radix, on skin inflammation: in vivo regulation of inflammation-associated gene expression. *Biochem Pharmacol.* 2003 Oct 1;66(7):1271–8.

Choi YK, Han IK, Yoon HK. Ipriflavone for the treatment of osteoporosis. *Osteoporos Int.* 1997;7 Suppl 3:S174–8.

Conney AH, Lysz T, Ferraro T, Abidi TF, Manchand PS, Laskin JD, Huang MT. Inhibitory effect of curcumin and some related dietary compounds on tumor promotion and arachidonic acid metabolism in mouse skin. *Adv Enzyme Regul.* 1991;31:385–96.

Croce CM. How can we prevent cancer? *Proc Natl Acad Sci U S A.* 2001 Sep 25;98(20):10986–8.

Eldeen IM, Elgorashi EE, van Staden J. Antibacterial, anti-inflammatory, anticholinesterase and mutagenic effects of extracts obtained from some trees used in South African traditional medicine. *J Ethnopharmacol.* 2005 Oct 15.

Ernst E. Avocado-soybean unsaponifiables (ASU) for osteoarthritis: a systematic review. *Clin Rheumatol.* 2003 Oct;22(4–5):285–8.

Gennari C, Adami S, Agnusdei D, Bufalino L, Cervetti R, Crepaldi G, Di Marco C, Di Munno O, Fantasia L, Isaia GC, Mazzuoli GF, Ortolani S, Passeri M, Serni U,Vecchiet L. Effect of chronic treatment with ipriflavone in postmenopausal women with low bone mass. *Calcif Tissue Int.* 1997;61 Suppl 1:S19–22.

Gennari C, Agnusdei D, Crepaldi G, Isaia G, Mazzuoli G, Ortolani S, Bufalino L, Passeri M. Effect of ipriflavone—a synthetic derivative of natural isoflavones—on bone mass loss in the early years after menopause. *Menopause.* 1998 Spring;5(1):9–15.

Graf J. Herbal anti-inflammatory agents for skin disease. *Skin Therapy Lett.* 2000;5(4):3–5.

Halpner AD, Kellermann G, Ahlgrimm MJ, Arndt CL, Shaikh NA, Hargrave JJ, Tallas PG. The effect of an ipriflavone-containing supplement on urinary N-linked telopeptide levels in postmenopausal women. *J Womens Health Gend Based Med.* 2000 Nov;9(9):995–8.

Head KA. Ipriflavone: an important bone-building isoflavone. *Altern Med Rev.* 1999 Feb;4(1):10–22.

Hong T, Jin GB, Cho S, Cyong JC. Evaluation of the anti-inflammatory effect of baicalein on dextran sulfate sodium-induced colitis in mice. *Planta Med.* 2002 Mar;68(3):268–71.

Huang MT, Lysz T, Ferraro T, Abidi TF, Laskin JD, Conney AH. Inhibitory effects of curcumin on in vitro lipoxygenase and cyclooxygenase activities in mouse epidermis. *Cancer Res.* 1991 Feb 1;51(3):813–9.

Innes JF, Fuller CJ, Grover ER, Kelly AL, Burn JF. Randomised, double-blind, placebo-controlled parallel group study of P54FP for the treatment of dogs with osteoarthritis. *Vet Rec.* 2003 Apr 12;152(15):457–60.

Jantaratnotai N, Utaisincharoen P, Piyachaturawat P, Chongthammakun S, Sanvarinda Y. Inhibitory effect of Curcuma comosa on NO production and cytokine expression in LPS-activated microglia. *Life Sci.* 2005 Aug 15.

Joe B, Lokesh BR. Role of capsaicin, curcumin and dietary n-3 fatty acids in lowering the generation of reactive oxygen species in rat peritoneal macrophages. *Biocheim Biophys Acta.* 1994 Nov 10;1224(2):255–63.

Joe B, Rao UJ, Lokesh BR. Presence of an acidic glycoprotein in the serum of arthritic rats: modulation by capsaicin and curcumin. *Mol Cell Biochem.* 1997 Apr;169(1–2):125–34.

Katase K, Kato T, Hirai Y, Hasumi K, Chen JT. Effects of ipriflavone on bone loss following a bilateral ovariectomy and menopause: a randomized placebo-controlled study. *Calcif Tissue Int.* 2001 Aug;69(2):73–7.

Kumar V, Lewis SA, Mutalik S, Shenoy DB, Venkatesh, Udupa N. Biodegradable microspheres of curcumin for treatment of inflammation. *Indian J Physiol Pharmacol.* 2002 Apr;46(2):209–17.

Lequesne M, Maheu E, Cadet C, Dreiser RL. Structural effect of avocado/soybean unsaponifiables on joint space loss in osteoarthritis of the hip. *Arthritis Rheum.* 2002 Feb;47(1):50–8.

Li BQ, Fu T, Gong WH, Dunlop N, Kung H, Yan Y, Kang J, Wang JM. The flavonoid baicalin exhibits anti-inflammatory activity by binding to chemokines. *Immunopharmacology.* 2000 Sep;49(3):295–306.

Li FQ, Wang T, Pei Z, Liu B, Hong JS. Inhibition of microglial activation by the herbal flavonoid baicalein attenuates inflammation-mediated degeneration of dopaminergic neurons. *J Neural Transm.* 2005 Mar;112(3):331–47.

Li RW, Myers SP, Leach DN, Lin GD, Leach G. A cross-cultural study: anti-inflammatory activity of Australian and Chinese plants. *J Ethnopharmacol.* 2003 Mar;85(1):25–32.

Lim BO. Efficacy of wogonin in the production of immunoglobulins and cytokines by mesenteric lymph node lymphocytes in mouse colitis induced with dextran sulfate sodium. *Biosci Biotechnol Biochem.* 2004 Dec;68(12):2505–11.

Lim GP, Chu T, Yang F, Beech W, Frautschy SA, Cole GM. The curry spice curcumin reduces oxidative damage and amyloid pathology in an Alzheimer transgenic mouse. *J Neurosci.* 2001 Nov 1;21(21):8370–7.

Lin CC, Shieh DE. The anti-inflammatory activity of Scutellaria rivularis extracts and its active components, baicalin, baicalein and wogonin. *Am J Chin Med.* 1996;24(1):31–6.

Maheu E, Mazieres B, Valat JP, Loyau G, Le Loet X, Bourgeois P, Grouin JM, Rozenberg S. Symptomatic efficacy of avocado/soybean unsaponifiables in the treatment of osteoarthritis of the knee and hip: a prospective, randomized, double-blind, placebo-controlled, multi-center clinical trial with a six-month treatment period and a two-month follow-up demonstrating a persistent effect. *Arthritis Rheum.* 1998 Jan;41(1):81–91.

Makita K, Ohta H. Ipriflavone in the treatment of osteoporosis. *Nippon Rinsho.* 2002 Mar;60 Suppl 3:359–64.

Mihara R, Barry KM, Mohammed CL, Mitsunaga T. Comparison of antifungal and antioxidant activities of Acacia mangium and A. auriculiformis heartwood extracts. *J Chem Ecol.* 2005 Apr;31(4):789–804.

Minaguchi J, Koyama Y, Meguri N, Hosaka Y, Ueda H, Kusubata M, Hirota A, Irie S, Mafune N, Takehana K. Effects of ingestion of collagen peptide on collagen fibrils and glycosaminoglycans in Achilles tendon. *J Nutr Sci Vitaminol* (Tokyo). 2005 Jun;51(3):169–74.

Naik GH, Priyadarsini KI, Satav JG, Banavalikar MM, Sohoni DP, Biyani MK, Mohan H. Comparative antioxidant activity of individual herbal components used in Ayurvedic medicine. *Phytochemistry.* 2003 May;63(1):97–104.

Nakajima T, Imanishi M, Yamamoto K, Cyong JC, Hirai K. Inhibitory effect of baicalein, a flavonoid in Scutellaria Root, on eotaxin production by human dermal fibroblasts. *Planta Med.* 2001 Mar;67(2):132–5.

Ohta H, Komukai S, Makita K, Masuzawa T, Nozawa S. Effects of 1-year ipriflavone treatment on lumbar bone mineral density and bone metabolic markers in postmenopausal women with low bone mass. *Horm Res.* 1999;51(4):178–83.

Park BK, Heo MY, Park H, Kim HP. Inhibition of TPA-induced cyclooxygenase-2 expression and skin inflammation in mice by wogonin, a plant flavone from Scutellaria radix. *Eur J Pharmacol.* 2001 Aug 10; 425(2):153–7.

Pearn J. Acacias and aesculapius. Australian native wattles and the doctors they commemorate. *Med J Aust.* 1993 Dec 6–20;159(11–12):729–38.

Petrella RJ. Hyaluronic acid for the treatment of knee osteoarthritis: long-term outcomes from a naturalistic primary care experience. *Am J Phys Med Rehabil.* 2005 Apr;84(4):278–83; quiz 284, 293.

Piao HZ, Jin SA, Chun HS, Lee JC, Kim WK. Neuroprotective effect of wogonin: potential roles of inflammatory cytokines. *Arch Pharm Res.* 2004 Sep;27(9):930–6.

Saleem A, Ahotupa M, Pihlaja K. Total phenolics concentration and antioxidant potential of extracts of medicinal plants of Pakistan. *Z Naturforsch* [C]. 2001 Nov–Dec;56(11–12):973–8.

Schelonka EP, Usher A. Ipriflavone and osteoporosis. *JAMA.* 2001 Oct 17;286(15):1836–7.

Sham JS, Chiu KW, Pang PK. Hypotensive action of Acacia catechu. *Planta Med.* 1984 Apr;50(2):177–80.

Snibbe JC, Gambardella RA. Treatment options for osteoarthritis. *Orthopedics.* 2005 Feb;28(2 Suppl):s215–20.

Srivastava KC, Mustafa T. Ginger (Zingiber officinale) and rheumatic disorders. *Med Hypotheses.* 1989 May;29(1):25–8.

Srivastava KC, Mustafa T. Ginger (Zingiber officinale) in rheumatism and musculoskeletal disorders. *Med Hypotheses.* 1992 Dec;39(4):342–8.

Surh YJ, Chun KS, Cha HH, Han SS, Keum YS, Park KK, Lee SS. Molecular mechanisms underlying chemopreventive activities of anti-inflammatory phytochemicals: down-regulation of COX-2 and iNOS through suppression of NF-kappa B activation. *Mutat Res.* 2001 Sep 1;480–481:243–68.

Swarnakar S, Ganguly K, Kundu P, Banerjee A, Maity P, Sharma AV. Curcumin regulates expression and activity of matrix metalloproteinases 9 and 2 during prevention and healing of indomethacin-induced gastric ulcer. *J Biol Chem.* 2005 Mar 11;280(10):9409–15.

Wu JH, Tung YT, Wang SY, Shyur LF, Kuo YH, Chang ST. Phenolic antioxidants from the heartwood of Acacia confusa. *J Agric Food Chem.* 2005 Jul 27;53(15):5917–21.

Yang X, Thomas DP, Zhang X, Culver BW, Alexander BM, Murdoch WJ, Rao MN, Tulis DA, Ren J, Sreejayan N. Curcumin Inhibits Platelet-Derived Growth Factor-Stimulated Vascular Smooth Muscle Cell Function and Injury-Induced Neointima Formation. *Arterioscler Thromb Vasc Biol.* 2005 Oct 20.

Yu H, Ong B. Photosynthesis and antioxidant enzymes of phyllodes of Acacia mangium. *Plant Sci.* 2000 Oct 16;159(1):107–115.

Zautra AJ, Yocum DC, Villanueva I, Smith B, Davis MC, Attrep J, Irwin M. Immune activation and depression in women with rheumatoid arthritis. *J Rheumatol.* 2004 Mar;31(3):457–63.

# CHAPTER 6
# PUTTING IT ALL TOGETHER: THE FLEXCARE PROGRAM

Ades PA, Savage PD, Cress ME, Brochu M, Lee NM, Poehlman ET. Resistance training on physical performance in disabled older female cardiac patients. *Med Sci Sports Exerc.* 2003 Aug;35(8):1265–70.

Blumenthal JA, Emery CF, Madden DJ, George LK, Coleman RE, Riddle MW, McKee DC, Reasoner J, Williams RS. Cardiovascular and behavioral effects of aerobic exercise training in healthy older men and women. *J Gerontol.* 1989 Sep;44(5):M147–57.

Boyle CA, Sayers SP, Jensen BE, Headley SA, Manos TM. The effects of yoga training and a single bout of yoga on delayed onset muscle soreness in the lower extremity. *J Strength Cond Res.* 2004 Nov;18(4):723–9.

DiBenedetto M, Innes KE, Taylor AG, Rodeheaver PF, Boxer JA, Wright HJ,

Kerrigan DC. Effect of a gentle Iyengar yoga program on gait in the elderly: an exploratory study. Arch Phys Med Rehabil. 2005 Sep;86(9):1830–7.

Galantino ML, Bzdewka TM, Eissler-Russo JL, Holbrook ML, Mogck EP, Geigle P, Farrar JT. The impact of modified Hatha yoga on chronic low back pain: a pilot study. Altern Ther Health Med. 2004 Mar–Apr;10(2):56–9.

Harinath K, Malhotra AS, Pal K, Prasad R, Kumar R, Kain TC, Rai L, Sawhney RC. Effects of Hatha yoga and Omkar meditation on cardiorespiratory performance, psychologic profile, and melatonin secretion. J Altern Complement Med. 2004 Apr;10(2):261–8.

Parshad O. Role of yoga in stress management. West Indian Med J. 2004 Jun;53(3):191–4.

Raub JA. Psychophysiologic effects of Hatha Yoga on musculoskeletal and cardiopulmonary function: a literature review. J Altern Complement Med. 2002 Dec;8(6):797–812.

# Index

## RECIPES INDEX

## ABOUT THE AUTHOR

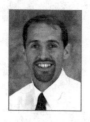

Shawn M. Talbott, Ph.D., is trained in sports medicine, health management, exercise physiology and nutritional biochemistry. He is the recipient of a dozen competitive research awards and has published over 100 articles on nutrition, health and fitness. In addition, Dr. Talbott has consulted for numerous athletic teams and organizations, including the Utah Jazz and the U.S. Track and Field Association. He lives near Salt Lake City, Utah.